THE
CLOSEST
of
STRANGERS

THE
CLOSEST
of
STRANGERS

JAMES JUDGE, M.D.

WORD PUBLISHING
NASHVILLE
A Thomas Nelson Company

Published by Word Publishing, a Thomas Nelson, Inc., company, P.O. Box 141000, Nashville, Tennessee 37214.

Scripture quotations are from the King James Version of the Bible.

ISBN 0-8499-1665-8 (hardcover)

Printed in the United States of America

For Cindy . . . stranger no more.

"Often, often, often, goes the Christ in the stranger's guise."

—OLD CELTIC POEM

CONTENTS

ACKNOWLEDGMENTS

There are many people to whom I must render heart-felt thanks.

To my literary agent, Bruce Barbour, who broke what is undoubtedly the first rule of being a literary agent—never take on a first-time author. Thank you for your cheerleading and for all you did to convince publishers to look at the manuscript.

To everyone who worked on this project at Word Publishing, for making the experience so seamless and enjoyable. Special thanks to Bridgett O'Lannerghty for her fine editing, and to Ami McConnell for her design and management skills, turning the manuscript into a beautiful book. And to Mark Sweeney, whose faith in this project was unbending. If there is a message in this book it is in large part due to Mark's encouragement to just say it.

To my daughters, Emily, Katie, and Jenny. Your encouragement and love are a constant grace in my life.

To my wife, Cindy, who saw this book coming from a distance. Your gift of faith continues to work magic in my life twenty-five years later. Short of pen to paper, you are more responsible for this work becoming a reality than anyone else.

And finally, to the patients who allowed me the unspeakable privilege of walking with them for a time, my most humble thanks.

INTRODUCTION

A few years ago, I had the privilege of hearing Nobel laureate Elie Wiesel address a room full of writers. Mr. Wiesel paused as he looked out over a crowded gymnasium and then delivered two succinct pieces of advice to those who would write:

> Write only if you cannot live without writing.
> Write only what you alone can write.

I felt his words resonate in my soul, and I think his advice best sums up what has motivated this book. These pages contain an anthology of true stories. With some of the stories I have changed certain identifying information in order to protect the confidentiality of the patients. They are written as remembered, without going back to clarify details, because I was afraid that if I did it would alter the impact the stories have had on me. And quite frankly, going back to clarify the details is not a luxury life usually affords us. Some of the stories have had a gestation period of nearly twenty years. I wrote early versions of them as a medical student, and at the time I could not have told you why I wrote them, only that I had to. Capturing them with words helped me deal with what I was facing and participating in and being formed by each day. Writing was both a form of release and a means of getting at least a partial hold on what was happening inside me as a result of my part in the stories. It was letting go and grabbing on for dear life all at the same time. It was my best therapy.

These are the stories of my intimate strangers. Faces that have haunted me and, I suppose, haunt me still. People I barely knew, but in some ways came to know more deeply than those with whom they had shared their entire lives. Maybe more deeply than I knew myself. With them I shared a privileged moment or a string of moments over a span of months or years, moments that were often supercharged with what felt like unjustified intimacy. At times it was as if I had stumbled into someone else's confessional. I squirmed and sweated, feeling I had not earned the right to hear what I was hearing—stories of striving with life and God and love and sex and death and seemingly everything except the sore throat or the headache or the fatigue written in my appointment book. You can spend a lifetime with someone and never get around to talking about these kinds of things. Over the years I learned that sometimes the opposite is also true—you can squeeze life's most crucial questions into fifteen- and twenty- and thirty-minute slots. Maybe it's the compression that generates the heat.

When asked what this book was going to be about, at first I had a hard time coming up with an answer. All I knew was that inside me there were these stories struggling for birth, and it was only after they were born that I saw they bore a certain family resemblance. I think what binds these stories together, and probably binds me to the stories, is that ultimately they are eyewitness accounts of the action of grace in the lives of my patients and, in a very real sense, my own life. They are accounts of grace's ruthless incursion into the dark spaces in our lives, the places more often characterized by fear and isolation and pain and at least the thin shadow of death, the unavoidable places through which none of us want to travel. Especially alone. Foreign territory that, at first glance, seems to harbor anything but grace.

And yet in each story, as it began to form on the page, I realized that what I had witnessed, more than anything else, was a certain grace. Certain in the sense of peculiar, unique, and personal. Certain in the sense of undeniable and always there. As I wrote the stories—or maybe in a truer sense, they wrote themselves—it seemed to me that each of them was like one of those Magic Eye dotted pictures, where if you stare long enough and hard enough, you begin to see another picture . . . buried, imbedded, hidden somewhere deeply within the first. One that initially seems to have no apparent connection to the one from which it springs. A dolphin jumps out at you from a picture of the New York skyline. A foolish clown materializes out of a mountain landscape. The first picture is flat and fuzzy, while the imbedded picture is three-dimensional and full of motion. One is obvious; the other you have to learn to look for, almost to the point of going fuzzy yourself. And oddly enough, that second picture is sometimes most easily seen when you aren't looking for it at all.

It was this second picture, this picture of an always-present, absurd grace that drew me to these stories and linked them together. Each one is a different rendering of God in action. With some of them it was obvious, clear, and simple. It popped out at me right away. Other times it was subtle, surprising me, standing quietly close by; like an old friend who comes from a long way off and, smiling, waits there in the crowd for you to recognize his face. It often came disguised, sometimes hideously, sometimes bizarrely. Like the clown in the landscape, out of nowhere, suddenly standing on his head, blowing me a big raspberry. Maybe just to make sure I didn't miss the point.

I was a witness to grace for sure, but not always a willing one. I was a player, like it or not, caught up in the drama of these people's lives by the simple act of listening. And try as I did early on to pretend that my white coat could protect me from their hurting and absurdity and joy and tragedy, I eventually saw that coat for what it really was—less armor, more costume. Something that simply identified my place in the play—nothing more, nothing less.

There are many in medicine today who would caution physicians about the dangers that come with letting their patients touch them emotionally. I think, for the most part, they are wrong. What they fail to see is an even greater danger—the danger inherent in disconnecting. The risk of missing the gift that comes with opening your heart. More than anything else, it is the gift of becoming more completely human, more like what we were intended to be. Frederick Buechner has said that he believes there is really only one plot to all our stories. And this is it: God, using our lives and the world and one another, conspires to make us all into Christs in one way or another, all into healers. Sometimes with our cooperation, often times without it. It is that thread that runs through the narrative of these stories; how in the course of the paths we took together, we helped each other become just a little more human in the fullest and most glorious and God-inspired use of that word. I believe it is, in the end, the only story worth telling.

TIMMY AND MARK

The first thing I saw when I woke up was the large schoolroom clock high up on the wall of the closet-like "on-call" sleeping room. 5:30 A.M. I closed my eyes and did the math. Last call was a little after three, which meant I'd managed two and a half hours of uninterrupted sleep. Not bad for pediatrics call. And the clock was still ticking. I rolled over and faced the window, and through one bleary half-opened eye, I watched the day begin. Outside, at the top of the hill, November's naked hardwoods stood black against a mouse-colored predawn sky. Slowly, imperceptibly, pinkish hues seeped into the gray background. The parallel slits of the window's wide-open venetian blinds made it look as if the entire scene had been mistakenly printed on a piece of lined composition paper, inviting someone to pick up a pen and begin to write that day's story. Although I wasn't quite sure of the plot, the main characters were already fixed in my mind: Timmy and Mark.

Timmy and Mark were two pediatric patients I cared for during my last year of medical school. Although in terms of personality they were about as different as two kids could be, the one talent they did have in common was their effortless ability to capture the hearts of those around them. They'd certainly captured mine. With Timmy, a five-year-old undergoing chemotherapy, I think what got to me was his crazy, almost brazen disregard for all the fearful and frightening things that swirled around him. With Mark, an eight-year-old with a chronic lung condition, what melted me most was the wide-eyed fear he just couldn't seem to shake. Looking back now I wonder if, as opposite as they were, those two children weren't in some way a mirror in which I saw my own confused reflection.

Mark had a severe lung disease called cystic fibrosis. One of the things this condition does is cripple a child's ability to fight off infection. Mark's life so far had been a sequence of one infection cascading into another, resulting in severe damage to his lungs. In recent years there have been many breakthroughs in the treatment of cystic fibrosis, but twenty years ago there was comparatively little we could do for these kids. We treated their pneumonias and bronchial infections with antibiotics and did a lot of aggressive respiratory therapy, and more than anything else we just hoped. Hoped that tomorrow would not bring with it the runny nose that might work itself into a cough, a cough that could then complicate into a pneumonia, a pneumonia we might or might not be able to treat.

Getting close to Mark became a crusade with me, but it was a hard go. Mark had been hospitalized fifteen to twenty times, and somewhere in that process he lost something—a child's unchallenged readiness to expect good things and just enjoy "today." I think Mark expected his today would probably be like a lot of his yesterdays, full of scary things. Scary food and scary smells and scary machines and scary people. It was with people that he really turned on the caution lights. Mark had watched a whole assembly line of "best buddy" doctors and nurses blaze into his life like sparklers, then just as suddenly as they had appeared, burn out and fade away. It left him leery of forming quick attachments to anyone in a white coat.

Mark would sit in his bed, mostly being careful. Careful not to wrinkle the sheets, careful to say "please and thank you, sir and ma'am," careful even of how he moved. Really careful about who he let in. He was always freshly scrubbed, his short brown hair strictly combed and parted, and his room was always militarily neat and in good order. The scene made me wonder if he was bucking for an early release on good behavior. As you talked to him, his large black-brown eyes remained on alert, looking both at you and through you, as if he were on never-ending sentry duty. I could never seem to get Mark to let down, and it frustrated me. I wanted to talk to him, really talk to him. Tell him it was okay to relax a little bit. Tell him we weren't going to take off any points for wrinkling the sheets. Tell him he wasn't the only one around here who was afraid. But nothing seemed to work. He dragged the fear around with him everywhere he went.

The world had conspired and robbed him of one of childhood's true distinctives, the capacity for trust. It had evaporated way too soon. In some ways what I saw sitting so carefully in that bed was not a child at all, but a small adult imprisoned in a child's realm of no control. What was it like to be locked in a world so full of the incomplete and incomprehensible? A world where you just took direction. Where everyone else seemed to know everything and you knew nothing and were just supposed to sit and go along with it all. Sometimes I wondered whether what touched me most about Mark was how alike at times our worlds really were.

Timmy, on the other hand, was Mark's alter ego. He was a happy Tasmanian devil, threatening to spin out of control at any moment. For him the hospital was one big game board, a blown-up version of Candy Land or Chutes and Ladders. He was uncontainable, especially physically, to the great dismay of the nursing staff. Nurses, as a group, tend to be pretty anal retentive and view obedience to rules and schedules as the greatest of godly virtues. Timmy took a distinctly different view. He saw the rules more like a set of monkey bars placed there for his personal pleasure. Swinging from them upside down and laughing was his greatest joy. In the midst of his chronic disobedience, Timmy would just stand there, on the rare occasions he just stood anywhere, and dare you not to love him. He was a five-year-old little boy who somehow, by some miracle, did not appreciate the gravity of his situation. He had a form of childhood leukemia and was in the middle of his third round of chemotherapy. His chances of survival were just about fifty-fifty.

Nothing seemed to intimidate him. Timmy was undaunted by both his illness and his physical appearance. He was a study in contrast. He was chronically pale with dark circles under large blue-blue twinkling eyes. His normally blond hair was reduced to that typical postchemo dandelion fluff, what little was left threatening to blow away with the next breeze. This made his face ageless, and when you looked at him, it was as if you saw him at five and fifteen and eighty-five all at the same moment. Nothing slowed him down. He tore about the pediatric floor with abandon, his pint-size hospital gown flowing all around him, continually flashing bystanders with either his Big Bird undies or, on the days when he decided undies were optional, his own anatomy through the gown's always-open back door.

This of course kept the nurses' own undies in a perpetual bundle. For fear of having him end up on the roof or in the street or up the flagpole, they established a schedule (what else?) where some nursing student or medical student or other unpaid peon was assigned to be with Timmy every hour until his battery ran down around seven o'clock at night.

I drew the 4–5 P.M. shift, which worked out great because that was when the local TV channel played back-to-back reruns of *The Little Rascals*. We made a game out of it. At four o'clock Timmy and I would race to his room, get the chairs set up side by side theater-style, turn on the TV, and, since Timmy's and my sense of humor were at about the same developmental stage, laugh ourselves silly. It was about the only continuous hour that he sat anywhere (between commercials of course). Timmy could easily have been a character on *The Little Rascals* himself. There was almost no mischief we watched that I think Timmy did not find both inviting and worth imitating. I don't think the nurses ever caught on to how much of his craziness had its creative origin in that particular time slot.

I loved watching Timmy during the shows. His shabby

exterior only accentuated the bundle of life within. The contrast between how he looked outside and who he was inside nearly broke my heart. Part of me wanted to put my arm around him, to protect him, to warn him of the dangers that lurked all around. The side effects of the chemotherapy and the possible germs hiding behind every visitor, every mask. On the other hand, I realized that childhood and foolishness and not knowing were for him particular blessings. His innate ability to trust was a strong armor. He never had to deal with all the terrible "what ifs" that assault and paralyze adults. He was locked into today and for Timmy, unlike Mark, today looked pretty darn good. The hospital was one giant playground where the refrigerators were stocked with plenty of ice cream and there was always someone to hang out with.

I was doing a two-month-long pediatric subinternship and had both Timmy and Mark on my service. A subintern functions like an intern, which means that for day-to-day patient-care decisions, I was the first person called. Although there was a senior pediatric resident and a staff pediatrician looking over my shoulder, I felt for the first time a feeling that would become an enduring part of my daily world: the overwhelming sense of responsibility. Good or bad, I believed that whatever happened to those two kids during my watch was my burden to bear.

Because it was my last year, I was caught in the throes of trying to decide what kind of doctor I was going to be, and this rotation was designed to help me make that decision. I had already made part of the decision. I wasn't destined to be a surgeon. The surgeons I had been with on my surgery rotation all had a self-confidence that bordered on arrogance. The emphasis on procedures also grated against something very basic inside me. It wasn't Mrs. Smith in Room 112, it was "the gallbladder" or "the appendix" or "the hemorrhoid." The patient interaction was missing, and that was the part, even then, that I loved the most.

I went through the same schizophrenic process with each of my other primary-care rotations. When I was on medicine, I wanted to be an internist. When I was on obstetrics, I wanted to deliver babies. I loved pediatrics, and I could even see myself as a psychiatrist. I suppose it really shouldn't have been a surprise that I ended up choosing an old specialty with a new name, family practice. In a way it was a nondecision that somehow reinforced my own ongoing delusion that I could do it all. Maybe that was my own brand of arrogance.

I took an almost automatic dislike to the senior pediatric resident. He just didn't fit my image of what a doctor was supposed to be like. He was tall, lanky, with a dark, scraggly wannabe beard. He had a chronic disheveled look that made me wonder if he had slept in his clothes, and even on those rare occasions that he did manage to scare up a tie, he still looked like a homeless guy pretending to be a doctor. A two-inch chewed-up toy bear afflicted with "the dreaded mange" clung desperately to his stethoscope, and his white coat was always stained with something unidentifiable, something you just hoped was mustard. When it came to his interaction with the rest of the care team, he preferred the image of a hard guy, which struck me as vaguely humorous. It was like James Cagney trying to be a pediatrician. How does that work? He was always eating something while we discussed the life-and-death aspects of the patients we were caring for, and in between chewing and swallowing, he felt obligated to toss in little editorial comments like, "We'll probably lose this one," or "This kid doesn't have a prayer."

"Yep, there's a darn good chance this kid isn't going to make it," he said, his leg draped over the back of a chair swinging disjointedly back and forth like a pendulum. "That chemo, man . . . it's a killer." He was talking about Timmy.

The combination of his careless macho medical talk and the ever-present aroma of peanut butter or banana, or whatever junk food du jour he'd just pulled from his bottomless lunch bag, kept me perpetually irritated. Whenever he started into his "Dr. Rambo" act, I found myself wincing as this balloon of panic grew bigger inside. It was almost as if I believed he would inadvertently cause a bad result simply by predicting it. I watched him, wanting him to just shut up. We were the captains of this team. We of all people shouldn't acknowledge the possibility of defeat. But he kept at it, and each time he did, it felt as if we were giving something up.

I guess I was still pretty idealistic about medicine, and his laissez-faire attitude seemed almost sacrilegious. First of all, how could he talk like that? Where was the reverence for what we were doing? We weren't talking about some far-emoved case. We were talking about a child, somebody's child, a human being not fifty feet down the hall. It would take me years to recognize this often-employed false bravado on the part of doctors and nurses for what it really was: a smoke screen. A smoke screen usually employed by someone who shared all the same feelings that churned inside of me, someone just as clueless as I was about what to do with them. We were both, in our own ways, playing the same game of self-defense, working hard to put some distance between ourselves and the hurt. His method was pretending to be unaffected. Refusing to acknowledge even the possibility that something bad might happen was mine. I guess we were just wearing camouflage of a slightly different color.

Mark and Timmy were definitely the two sickest children on the peds floor and seemed to be on polar-opposite courses, as if they were involved in a deadly game of tug of war. If Timmy lost ground, Mark gained it. If Timmy had a good day—his blood counts up, his fever down—Mark seemed to go the other direction. If Mark's breathing was improving then Timmy would run a temperature. I watched their give and take and wondered who would get dragged first across the dark pit that stood between them.

The answer came sooner than I expected. Timmy scared us all with three days of spiking temperatures and low blood counts. I felt my own anxiety level tracing the ups and downs of his temperature graph. Either physically or mentally I spent most of my days with him. I was obsessed with his progress, convinced that I was single-handedly responsible for whatever happened to him. The pediatric resident watched me and I think, although I couldn't see it then, was motivated by concern for me.

"You got to watch out, Judge," he said, using a Mars bar as a lecture baton, having just missed the waste can with the crumpled wrapper from his third one that morning.

"You can't get too involved with these patients." Pointing

the candy bar at me for emphasis, he concluded, "It's not good for them and it's definitely not good for you."

I stood there staring at him, immediately rejecting what he said, mostly because it just felt wrong. Caring for patients had to mean more than knowing the right antibiotic or doing the right procedure. Caring meant caring—by definition didn't it have to affect you? Second, I rejected what he said because I had already labeled and pegged him. I saw people as pretty much one-dimensional at that point in my life; they were only what I thought of them. Good/bad. Smart/dumb. Either/or.

Timmy's fever spiked higher every day, and on the third afternoon of the fever, I found myself sitting with Timmy and his mother watching *The Little Rascals,* although it was mostly me doing the watching. Timmy lay in his bed listless, barely opening his eyes. When he did he would look up feebly toward the TV suspended from the ceiling, then slip back into that world where his fight was going on. What was left of his hair was sweated down flat against his head, painted into careless whirlpools that gave testimony to the violence churning just below the surface. His was an interior battleground, where good white blood cells fought cancerous ones with chemotherapy, a terrible weapon, whose backfire was itself sometimes life-threatening. I sat there watching him, trapped in the limbo between worry and prayer. Once he looked up to see Spanky and Buckwheat getting chased down an alley by a policeman. A weak smile stole briefly across his face. Then his eyes closed, and he sank back below the surface one more time.

I went home late that night, leaving strict instructions to be called if anything changed. When I got home I gave my wife a brief report of the day. It was a brief report because my emotional language at that time consisted mostly of victories and conclusions, neither of which applied to what was actually going on with me right then. I left out the part about how scared I was, about how unprepared I felt for the human side of what I was dealing with. My medical school training, by its very structure, had sent a clear message about what's important and what's not. The road to becoming a doctor begins with two years of books. You are buried under a mountain of data, and somehow by cramming your head full of facts for two years you are supposed to be prepared for a lifetime on the front lines of humanity. As I lay there in bed that night, I was gripped with a panicked feeling that I had somehow missed a crucial class. What happened to the course about what it meant to be human? I should have been reading Dostoevsky alongside my cardiology text, and Brahms should have been mixed with biochemistry. But there was nothing like this. There was only silence on the topic, and by that silence a quiet acquiescence that an understanding of either human beings or myself was not essential.

I got up at 5:30 the next morning, showered, and rushed back up to the pediatric ward. I went straight to Timmy's room but found it empty. My heart sank. I looked down the hall and saw the night clerk and the day clerk going through the changing of the guard. "Tell me something happened to him last night and no one called me. Just tell me," I muttered to myself. I was panicked inside, fear blurring into anger. As I started back toward the nursing station, I noticed Timmy's name on a room across the hall. Could they have moved him?

I poked my head in and just stood there staring, not believing it was real. There was Timmy, sitting up. Although weak and a little worse for the wear, the sparkle was definitely back. His mom was just stepping out of the bathroom, drying her hands.

"His fever broke late last night, and just as soon as it did he started waking up," she said, managing a cautious smile, a little worse for the wear herself.

Inside I felt a need to cry or dance or do a lot of things I didn't do, but something in my eyes must have betrayed me because Timmy's mom grabbed my arm and looked at me and said, "That was closer than I thought I could take." Then she paused a moment and simply said, "Thank you."

I looked over at Timmy and said reflexively, "He's a tough kid, Mrs. Thompson. Thank Timmy."

Or thank God, or thank the medicine or the luck of the draw, but whatever you do, don't thank me. But I think I missed the point entirely. I don't think she was thanking me for anything I had done medically. I think she was thanking me for caring, for standing with them, for putting my heart just a little bit in harm's way. All at once, the fact Timmy had made it through made the reality of what it would have been like if he hadn't all the more real, all the more frightening. It was a hooded, dark specter that stood and pointed its ghostly finger straight at me. As I thought about the last three days and the part I had played, all I could see was the paralyzing fear and the unanswered question: What would I have done if we had lost him? I thought back to the advice the pediatric resident had given me about getting too close. Maybe there was some sense in it after all.

As Timmy's course began to improve, Mark began to deteriorate. His breathing became progressively more labored and difficult. The respiratory treatments he received multiple times each day didn't seem to change anything. He began to spike high fevers and developed a severe pneumonia that our antibiotics didn't appear to touch. He was placed in an oxygen tent, which only seemed to remove him even further from us. He was more alone now than ever, a prisoner in a strange solitary world of cold damp swirling mist, boxed in a cruel cloud.

Mark's mother was omnipresent, a small round woman in her mid-to-late twenties whose manners made you think she was a good deal older. Her jet-black hair was pulled back tightly from her large muffin face, a small pair of wire-rimmed glasses resting precariously on her almost nonexistent nose. She wore nothing but sacklike home-sewn dresses, each a slightly modified version of the one before. There was never any appearance or mention of a father.

There was a grimness to her that seemed to penetrate deeper than the level of her son's illness. Her conversations with me were peppered with Bible verses that were used almost like magical incantations. Although my own faith journey had just barely begun, I couldn't escape feeling that she took the verses she so often quoted and used pieces of them to say whatever she needed them to say that day. I tried to talk to her about her faith and Mark's illness but it was difficult and awkward, as if she wasn't quite sure whether I was friend or foe. There seemed to be very little space to her religion. God controlled everything, but in some ways it seemed as if she controlled God, manipulating and backing him into a corner with his own promises. Almost like a genie in a bottle. Say a verse, rub the lamp, and presto chango, it all turns out the way you want.

I wasn't all that sure of exactly what I believed about faith and disease and healing. I knew God could heal if he chose to, but was he required to do so? Was faithlessness, as Mark's mother seemed to believe, the only reason he didn't do it more often? I wrestled with these questions alone. I could tell that expressing any form of doubt was a great sin in his mother's eyes and, sadly, no real dialogue ever developed between us. I mostly listened and watched. She spoke deliberately, her rural accent converting many one-syllable words to two syllables.

"Awell things work together for gooed, to those that love the Lored" was the ending to almost every encounter I had with her. Always said with an emphasis on the dependent clause at the end, always with a filmy smile that barely covered over the titanic struggle going on inside. It was a sword she used to fend off any bad news, a sword that became duller each day as her son's condition worsened. At times she turned this weapon on the doctors and nurses as well, as if we were all somehow causing her son's sickness by our own lack of faith, or a faith not exactly like hers. As Mark became more and more ill, his mother became more and more antagonistic.

She stood at his side like a palace guard whenever anyone came to see him. Her round gray eyes looked like ball bearings, and she set her face like flint, daring us to do anything. I was just confused. Whose side did she think we were on? Looking back now, I think the deep current of anger that flowed just beneath her surface was undeniable and it needed to go somewhere. It was probably just easier to direct it toward us than anywhere else.

The elders of her church came up one night when I was on call to pray for healing. Mark's mother invited me to stay. During it all, I felt the intensity of her steel eyes as she slipped me looks that seemed to say, "Just watch, now you'll see." The three leisure-suited elders with slicked-back hair took their places around Mark's bed. They smelled of peppermint and chewing tobacco. They laid their hands on Mark and began to pray. The problem was it didn't sound much like prayer, or at least the kind of prayer an eight-year-old kid needed. There was no sound of comfort here. The words felt severe, full of tension and frustration and an inescapable strain of blame.

"We KNOW, Lored, that if we only have faith as a mustard seed, we can move mountains," one of them barked.

"JESUS!" another cried out, startling me. I couldn't tell at first whether it was an exclamation or a curse. "Those little children long ago were healed because their parents had the FAITH to make them well. REMOVE this child's sickness from him. Give his mother the faith to make it so."

I knew I was supposed to be praying too, but I couldn't take my eyes off Mark lying almost motionless in the oxygen tent. Through the mist I could see his eyes were clenched tightly, but I couldn't tell whether he was taking it all in or shutting it all out.

Mark's breathing seemed to stabilize for a few days after that, but then he suddenly got much worse, and we were forced toward a decision no one wanted to make. He was

THE CLOSEST OF STRANGERS

getting too tired breathing on his own. He could barely open his eyes now and had to be moved and cared for almost as if he were unconscious. Our only other recourse was to intubate him and get him on a respirator. But this had definite dangers associated with it. Once on, it might be very difficult to get him off. There was a significant chance that his diseased and damaged lungs might never be able to work on their own again, and he could be stuck on the respirator forever. But there didn't seem to be any alternative. We were losing him by inches every day. We talked to Mark's mother. Her reaction was predictable—we had become the enemy. She didn't want any of our machines. Mark would recover on his own; God would heal him. I cringed as she said it, caught somewhere between my own lack of faith and fear for hers, afraid of the inevitable breakdown to come.

The next morning Mark had a severe coughing episode and turned blue. Quick action by the respiratory therapist brought him back to some level of stability. His mother witnessed it all and was terrified. The pediatric attending physician for Mark was a cystic fibrosis expert and knew Mark and his mother very well. She was a portly woman in her early sixties, an odd combination of brilliance and grandmother. Her ability to balance both the emotion and the expertise needed to care for these very sick children partially explained her legendary status at the medical center. She had cared for hundreds of patients with Mark's exact problem and had an uncanny ability to predict what direction a kid was going to take. Where Mark was concerned, she did not like the way the wind was blowing. I think she knew Mark's only hope, if he had any at all, was on that respirator. He just couldn't keep at it much longer. She decided to strike while the emotion of it all was still fresh. She sat down with Mark's mom alone in a little alcove off the ward's empty playroom and came back twenty minutes later with a signed release to place him on the respirator.

In a hurried voice, she told me, "Jim, call the ICU and tell them we're moving him down right away . . . before she changes her mind. I'll talk with anesthesia."

In a strange way getting his mother to sign the papers felt both victorious and deceptive at the same time. We had taken advantage of her fear. Whether it was an unfair advantage or not, I didn't know. Maybe it didn't even matter. We were acting on Mark's behalf to the best of our medical knowledge. His mother would have to resolve her own faith questions at a later date.

Within the hour Mark was moved to the intensive care unit, where an anesthesiologist sedated him, intubated him, and put him on a respirator. Mark barely moved now, as if everything he had was directed to just getting the next breath in and out. I was unschooled in the whole respirator thing, but I could tell by the emotional tone of the conversation between the head of anesthesia and the pediatric attending that we were walking a tightrope. The pediatric resident took me aside and interpreted for me.

"Anesthesia's all uptight. The kid is doing worse by the hour. It's taking too much pressure to keep him oxygenated. They're worried we'll blow a lung or something." He stood in front of Mark's bed just shaking his head. "That kid collapses a lung and it's all over," he whispered to me in hushed tones. Despite his vernacular, I thought I caught a glimmer of something I hadn't seen in this guy before, something close to real concern.

As if realizing he'd momentarily let his mask slip, he quickly added in a false sort of "poor me" tone. "And wouldn't you know it. I'm on call. Oh well, I guess I know where I'm going to be all night."

Mark's condition continued to deteriorate. Hour by hour there was more machine and less child in his cubicle. Late the next afternoon, while we were all in the intensive care unit, his heart rate suddenly sank to a third of its normal rate, and his already-poor skin color turned dark and dusky.

"Oh God, he's arresting; I think he blew his lung," yelled the resident. We got Mark's struggling mother and her pastor out of the way into a different corner of the unit, yanked the curtain around his bed and began resuscitation. The next hour was a disjointed montage of x-rays and chest tubes and blood sampling all happening at the same time, seven of us all frantically doing something we hoped would help. But it was a losing battle. Mark's heart rate sank lower and lower no matter what we did. We started chest compressions alternating with his respirator, but it was useless. After almost forty minutes of everything we could do, the pediatric attending physician stepped back from Mark's bed, paused a moment, then finally looked at us all and said, "I think it's over. Thank you, everyone, for your efforts." I stood there horror stricken. It had never occurred to me we could lose. It was the first time I had ever seen a child die.

Mark's mother read our faces as we came out from behind the curtain, already knowing the answer to the question she couldn't possibly ask. The pediatric attending walked slowly over to her, gently took her two hands, and told her Mark was gone. For a moment she didn't move. She just looked confused, as if the doctor was speaking a terrible language she did not understand. Then she collapsed into the arms of her pastor who tried awkwardly to console her, but even he had no words.

The nurses did what they needed to do, then let Mark's mother and her pastor come back behind the curtain to say good-bye to her son. As she approached the curtain, her walk was slow and hesitant, as if torn between almost equal forces drawing her forward and pushing her back. The curtain was drawn behind them to give them some false sense of privacy, but it was useless. The emotion in the room made the curtain almost transparent. A thick and heavy quiet swept over the intensive care unit, a terrible anticipation that seemed to go on forever. Somehow it wasn't what I expected. Then, like a crack of lightning out of a clear sky, the silence was shattered with a desperate powerful voice, and I heard his mother scream out: "IN THE NAME OF JESUS, I COMMAND YOU, RISE UP!"

Time stopped. No one in the unit moved. Each of us was frozen in his place. Even the machines seemed to hold their breath. I felt the hair on the back of my neck stand up, almost as if someone were breathing close behind me.

Her voice called out once more, even louder, breaking this time with emotion.

"IN THE NAME . . . IN THE NAME OF THE LORD JESUS CHRIST, I COMMAND YOU, CHILD . . . RISE UP!"

Again, a smothering, sickening, deafening silence. The slow-motion sound of someone's world caving in. I stood there trembling, struggling to push back down whatever it was at that moment rising out of the depths of my own soul. Embarrassment and hope and despair and awe. But more than anything else, I stood engulfed in a choking cloud of longing, as if something I had wanted all my life stood just barely out of sight. Maybe it was a longing for everything I believed in to be shown to be undeniably true, for a miracle. Or maybe it was a longing for a faith like this, a faith that could compel you to put it all on the line in one final insane bet. Or maybe it was much simpler. Maybe what I longed for was nothing more than a happy ending, for this beautiful child to blink his eyes and just sit up. Whatever it was, the feeling of it was familiar. It felt strangely like homesickness.

The next sound from behind the curtain was a gradual crescendo of muffled sobs that seemed to echo on and on. A strange reverse echo that, instead of fading as it repeated, got louder each time it bounced off the surfaces of the ceiling and the machinery and our own hearts. Finally the curtain parted and, heavily supported by her pastor, Mark's mother slowly left the unit, oblivious to all of us who were powerless to do anything except watch her. As the door of the intensive care unit closed behind her, I wondered whether she had lost more than her son.

The peds resident and I exchanged a look. I steeled myself for some kind of crass comment, but he surprised me again. He looked quickly back down at the note he was writing on Mark's chart, working hard to wipe away the tears before anyone would notice.

Almost in a daze, I meandered slowly back up to the pediatric floor. It was after four o'clock, and *The Little*

Rascals had been on for ten minutes. I stood in the doorway of Timmy's room and looked in. He had already moved our two front-row seats into their positions. He was looking up at the screen, giggling, then he shot me an impatient smile that said, "Come on, you're late. You don't want to miss this."

I walked over and dropped down into the seat next to him and blankly watched the absurdity of these children caught in one continuous chase scene, oblivious to the hapless adults and the danger that seemed to stalk them everywhere. I put my arm around Timmy, and we sat there and together we began to laugh. I laughed much harder than I needed to. I laughed until I cried.

POSTSCRIPT

Timmy did well with his chemotherapy and was discharged from the hospital, and I moved on to another rotation. Four months later, while working in the E.R., I saw Timmy's name on the board and my heart sank. I was immediately sure he'd had a recurrence of his cancer. I found him tearing up the orthopedic room where his mother, smiling, reassured me they were just there to get his arm checked out. He had sprained his wrist beating up on his older brother. Some trick he learned from Spanky no doubt. She told me he was doing fine, his blood counts were normal, and it looked like he would make it. I never saw him again. As far as I know, she was right.

In the weeks that followed Mark's death, I was haunted by that moment in the ICU, when his mother called upon God to raise her son from the dead. I tried to sort out what I had witnessed that afternoon. Was it simply the spectacle of a desperate mother overwhelmed with grief and guilt? Or was it a moment of grace, a living metaphor, a shadow of something that would some day, in some way, fall across all our paths? I fought a strange sense of guilt that was hard to shake. Maybe I felt guilty for not sharing her confidence, for choosing to stand in the crowd that day with those who watched breathlessly as she worked the high wire of her own faith without benefit of a net. Maybe it was that I wanted so desperately for God to show up on cue, knowing how averse he is to command performances.

The questions piled up. Why Mark and not Timmy? Mark's mom was trusting in God. From where I stood I couldn't see that Timmy's parents were relying on anything other than the expertise of the medical center and a little good luck. Where did God go that afternoon? Was he not listening or just off somewhere with more important matters? Or was he at that moment, as I later became convinced, closer to us all than the very air we breathed? Was it his nearness I felt so distinctly? Was it him standing there behind me, gently whispering an answer to both her prayer and mine? An unexpected and gentle answer, an answer that was neither yes nor no. An answer more like "not now . . . later." And what answer had Mark's mom heard? Where was her faith now?

A partial answer to that question came several weeks after Mark's death, when a card from his mother arrived on the pediatric floor. It was deliberate and polite, thanking everyone for their kind care of her son. On the front of the card was an old-fashioned picture of Jesus bent over a little girl's bed, his hand on hers. At the bottom was a Bible reference along with the words *Talitha cumi*. That evening I looked up the reference in a Bible at home. They were Aramaic words, the words of Jesus as he raised a little girl from the dead: "Little lamb, arise."

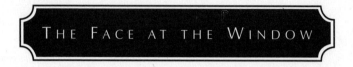

THE FACE AT THE WINDOW

I stepped out of my car, paused a moment and breathed in the cold morning air. There had been an early frost. It was one of those late September mornings when the cold north winds dip down into the Midwest, bringing with them a hint of what is to come. The sky looked almost too blue. It was nearly tangible, as if I could reach up and smear it like wet finger paint. I paused and looked at the ten-story hospital. I remember thinking that I, for one, was glad to be alive. I pulled on my white jacket and rushed across the parking lot to the front door.

I was a second-year family practice resident, which meant, essentially, that I had advanced from serf to indentured servant. I was halfway through a two-month cardiology rotation at this large community hospital, and part of my job was to do teaching rounds with the medical students who were also on my rotation. Things inside were already bustling—some patients coming in for outpatient work, others registering for admission, staff rushing everywhere. Everyone seemed to know exactly where they were going and were intent on getting there. The huge lumbering hospital was coming alive.

I was running a little late, so I hopped into the public elevator, which came more frequently than the staff and service elevators. I pressed 8 on the elevator keyboard and stepped back against the wall, and almost immediately regretted my decision—I had just become a curiosity on display. As people got on and off, they all went through the same routine. They looked at me in my white coat then immediately scanned the name on the jacket. What were my letters? Was I a lab tech or a medical student or a "real doctor"? Once they saw "MD" on the lapel, the look changed to one of strange expectancy, like I was supposed to start lecturing or sing or give the Disney tour. Tempting. I could do it like a big-top ringmaster.

"Ladies and gentlemen! Welcome to the amazing fourth floor, Psychiatry—troubled teens, anorexics, and men who wear ladies' lingerie. Next stop, Urology—kidney stones, sagging bladders, and other unmentionables."

It always made me squirm, as if I was somehow the one to blame for all the awkwardness in this little box of strangers. The silence remained as we all stared blankly forward, stealing furtive glances at one another, being carried floor by floor to our respective fates.

Each floor of the hospital had the same basic blueprint: three wings, connected to one another, by a large central nursing station. The public elevators let you off directly in front of the nursing station. The service elevators opened into a small linoleum-tiled room, which then opened through a pair of swinging doors into the middle wing of the hospital, just around the corner from the nursing station. Each of these service rooms had a large plate-glass window.

I got off the elevator on eight, the cardiology stepdown

unit, where patients are placed between their stay in the acute cardiac care unit and going home. It was a happy but tense floor: most everyone here was getting better, but most everyone here had definitely had the scare of their lives. It's a floor full of lifestyle changes and new resolutions. The two medical students in my charge were standing there waiting for me. They were typical early '80s types. Their hair was a little too long and their loose open shirts and wrinkled cords a little too casual. They had yet to learn that dressing well can buy patient confidence when your face is too young. Their short white coat pockets bulged with all the usual medical student paraphernalia: percussion hammers and otoscopes and, of course, the ever-present *Washington Manual*—the *Reader's Digest* abridged version of all medical knowledge. It is the official security blanket for America's doctors-in-waiting. They were big guys, both over six feet tall. One was an ex–college football player, thick and sturdy. The other was an ex-hippie, thin and poetic looking.

I looked at them and thought, *Well, at least they don't look like gunners.*

"Gunners" is a derogatory term used for students who are nearly rabid in the pursuit of their medical education. Sort of the marine recruits of the medical world. They are easy to spot. Too clean-cut, too academic, too slavish in their deference to authority. They are so far divorced from the human drama unfolding around them that it is almost comic. Their world tends to be textbook and two-dimensional. There is not much in their lives besides themselves and making the grade. It's as if they're continuously trying out for the team but in the process end up not really playing the game at all.

For them there is only one burning question: I wonder if this will be on the test?

I enjoyed teaching, but the whole system sometimes got to me. It was like one long fraternity initiation, the main theme of which was the denial of your own humanity. Gunners and technicians get rewarded while the humans are simply warned about the perils of being too soft. How strange that this most human of professions begins training its own children by first attempting to bleed any trace of humanity out of them. Maybe doctors can't teach doctors the secrets of the human heart. Maybe only patients can do that.

The two students greeted me smiling, but there was still that sense of fear in their expressions. It was a look I recognized because, in one way or another, we all shared it. More than anything else it was the fear of our own inadequacy, making all of us feel like impostors. It both bound us together and held us at arm's length. Deep down we all were sure of one thing—people believed there was more to us than was really there. Yet no one could be really honest and say, "You know, I don't know everything, but there are some things I've learned. Let's just do this together and pray to God that today, with whatever we face, it's enough." I am sure if anyone had said anything remotely like that anywhere during my medical training, the earth would have opened up and swallowed them whole, right then and there.

"Hello, gentlemen. I am Dr. Judge."

The words still felt weird as I said them, like I was pretending.

"Shall we begin."

We took an armload of charts and started down the hall,

going room to room. I had already familiarized myself with each of the cardiology service's patients, and my job now was to have the medical students examine each patient for pertinent physical findings, like distended neck veins or swollen ankles or heart murmurs. Then we would talk about the diagnosis, what that meant to the patient, and the best course of treatment. My teaching style was driven mostly by the personality of the students with me. Sometimes I presented the patient's case history much like the textbook, with all the pre-memorized sets of signs and symptoms. But if I picked up any know-it-all attitude from the students, I would lead them down any number of rabbit trails, forcing them to sort out the pertinent from the bizarre. This was probably more like real life. But these two guys seemed pretty fresh faced and up front. I decided to leave the humility lesson out of that morning's curriculum.

I always felt uncomfortable for the patient in the teaching process. It was hard to get over the gnawing sense that we were invading these people's privacy, maybe compromising their dignity just a little. Some of them, of course, loved it. I think it reinforced their own feelings of uniqueness and importance. Being poked and prodded somehow gave them a sense of worth—the more the merrier. What bothered me most, though, was that it felt like we didn't connect with them, as if the patients were merely props, teaching tools. But they weren't props, they were people. We weren't just standing in front of a "good" case of congestive heart failure, we were standing in front of a husband and an autoworker and a grandpa who was having trouble breathing and working and making love, and I wondered how his diagnosis affected the other parts of his life. It felt so clinical, so detached, as if we never got to the real issues—the ones that, although affected by the diagnosis, transcended it. How had the symptoms impacted this patient's hopes and dreams and fears? Why didn't we ever talk about this? Were we afraid of upsetting the patient, or was it just a screen for our own lack of answers? Maybe if we had had the courage to ask these kind of questions and really examine our patients in the fullest and deepest sense of that word, we would have been startled by how much we had in common with them.

While the students were busy examining the patients, I would pass the moments by leaning on the waist-high heating register that ran full length below the windows at the end of each room. I was drawn to the paint-box blue sky. It was so clear. I wanted to step right out into it. Freedom. To have a day where I could do whatever I wanted without a hundred people's expectations. I looked out over the trees and the city and the cars below, all moving fast to a somewhere I knew nothing about. Life was in full motion and it felt like I was missing it. What I didn't see as I went through this room-by-room ritual was the face of a man standing at the first window in the adjacent wing, staring out much like me. Not until it was too late.

We had worked our way back down the hall and were now in the patient room closest to the nursing station. I had just given the patient's history, and the two students with me were both bent over listening intently, trying to make themselves hear the subtle heart sounds I had described. I sat with my arms folded, waiting for them to finish listening to this patient's heart murmur so I could wax eloquent about its qualities and what it all meant and put the fear of God into them about the consequences of ever missing it. I was study-ing the patient's face, wondering to myself what he thought about all this, when I heard the first crash. I reflexively jumped away from the window, then took a step closer to it, unprepared in any way for what I saw. There was a man at the adjacent window of the other wing, ten feet away at most, frantically smashing the window again and again and again with a mop bucket. His eyes were blazing. He looked like a madman. The medical students both stepped away from the patient and toward the window. The three of us stood there in front of the large picture window, which had been trans-formed into our own personal life-size TV.

"What is he doing?" one of the medical students asked almost under his breath, as we all watched in disbelief. After crashing out most of the window, the man heaved the mop bucket out and then began to push the remaining shards of glass away with his bare hands. A wave of nausea swept over me as I started to realize his intentions. He kept look-ing over his shoulder, a look of desperate horror frozen on his face. I remember thinking it was not so much a horror of what was ahead of him, as of what was behind. There was something he was willing to pay any price to get away from. He looked terrorized, pursued, one step ahead of something monstrous, and he was doing everything in his power to escape. All in one moment, he leaned out the win-dow, struggled over the waist-high ledge, and then when he was halfway out, as if noticing us for the first time, he paused a moment and locked his eyes with mine. Then, arms at his side, he jumped headfirst.

"Oh God! Oh God! He jumped!" one of the medi-cal students screamed.

I caught my breath and rushed out of the room and around the elevators to the swinging doors opening into the service room from where he had jumped. My heart was beating wildly, and it took more courage than I knew I had to fling those doors open. Because of what I had seen on the man's face, I was sure there had to be someone else in that room, something that had pursued him, chased him out that window. Something unthinkable that I now had to face. I crashed through the doors. The room was cold and silent and, except for the broken glass and outside street sounds, empty.

I rushed to the window and looked down. I could see him lying six floors below on the roof of the pavilion that spanned the area between two of the wings of the hospital. He was crumbled like a discarded rag doll. I turned and ran straight into the medical students behind me.

"There's got to be a way onto that roof from the third floor," I shouted as I pushed them out of the way and rushed back into the hall where a crowd of employees and patients was forming. I screamed at the station clerk to call a code blue for the third floor and then slammed open the door to the stairway and began flying down the stairs four and five steps at a time, the medical students close on my heels. The race down felt like it would never end, and the whole way I was thinking, *What am I going to do? What am I going to do when I get there?* There is nothing in the *Washington Manual* about people jumping out of windows. When I got to the third floor I ran to the nursing station and between gasps asked if there was any way to get onto the pavilion's roof from this floor. The clerk was panicked and barely coherent. No one knew of any, so I ran into the first patient room to see if there was any way out through a window.

The room I ran into was a scene of hysteria. Three nurses were doing everything they could to get the two older bed-ridden women out of the room as fast as possible. The patients were hysterical, screaming, crying, "Help him! My God, why doesn't somebody help him?!" They were only acting out what was going on inside the rest of us. The bottom ledge of the patient windows on this floor was only two feet above the second-floor roof. The man who had jumped lay in a crumpled bleeding heap, not three feet outside their window. They had witnessed the impact because they had seen the falling glass, then his mop bucket, and then him. The nurses had the patient beds wedged in the entry of the room in their desperation to get the patients moved out, away from the grizzly sight outside their window. I climbed over the beds and tried to find some way of getting out onto that roof. The only opening was a two-foot-wide transom window that tilted open just halfway.

I turned to the medical students and yelled, "I think I can fit through there," and as if choreographed a hundred times before, they picked me up and inserted me in a single movement down through the transom, like a letter into a slot. The fit was tight and as I slid through all the buttons on the front of my shirt were ripped off. I found myself on my knees, with broken glass and gravel and blood all around. The panic and the screaming of a moment before were replaced with the final agonal breaths of the man at my knees and the soft, distant sounds of a city going about its business, not seeming to know or care. The man's arms and legs were arranged un-naturally, his eyes open and bulging but not seeing, his chest heaving deeply. I looked him over as best I could, and it was apparent that he had landed on his head. The entire back left portion of his skull was soft, indented. He had done the deed.

By now the medical students had also inserted the head nurse through the same window and we knelt together over the man.

"I don't think we have a lot to work with here, Sherri. This guy definitely landed on his head," I said, breathless.

"He's an employee, Jim. He works here," Sherri replied.

For the first time I looked at his face, really looked at it, and immediately recognized him. He worked maintenance. Or was it nursing? For some reason I thought I remembered him in postop with a stethoscope around his neck, taking vitals. But no, I must be wrong because I was sure I had seen him earlier that same week at about seven or eight o'clock in the evening. He was mopping the floor. Actually, he was just leaning on his mop. He had looked up and stared at me as I passed. He didn't say anything. Neither did I.

I had just walked by.

By this time his pupils were starting to dilate, and he began to slip away. Sherri and I looked at one another and knew we had to at least attempt a resuscitation, even though we were, at best, just going through the drill. The futility of it made us feel false. We started an IV. Support people handed equipment to us through the window. A respiratory therapist got out through the window as well, and we intubated the patient. The man's respiratory pattern was all but gone, and within minutes his pulse disappeared too. Someone handed me a pair of defibrillator paddles. We shocked him once, twice.

No response.

As my hands got him into position to transfer onto the backboard, I felt the soft mushy side of his skull and my stomach turned. We got him positioned and began doing chest compressions. We started CPR. One, two, three, four, five . . . breathe.

The high canyon walls of the hospital's two adjacent wings towered above us. The sun was shining on the other side of the building, casting a deep shadow on our side. It was eerie, like a place nobody had ever been before, like the dark side of the moon. As our resuscitation attempt continued, I became conscious of our audience. For ten floors up there were two or three faces clustered at almost every window, watching the real-life drama unfolding below. "So great a cloud of witnesses." It felt unreal, as if I were part of some morality play and this man in my arms was Everyman and the play was our own corporate story. The wind was whipping my shirt. It defied gravity, flying about me, the bright white T-shirt underneath stained with blood. We were on stage, locked in a kind of hand-to-hand combat. And even though everyone standing at their own box seat already suspected how it would end, the play went on and everyone continued to watch. I guess it's not the end that is ever really in question. And so we kept at it. The young doctor, the pretty nurse, battling the unbeatable foe, working desperately to save someone who sought another kind of salvation.

We were soon joined by two of the ER doctors who gained access to the roof by a hook and ladder that had been rushed over by the local fire department. The hospital-associated day-care class was out playing, and when they saw the fire engine pull up, the teacher brought a group of preschoolers over to get a closer look at the fire truck. When the teacher realized there was a real-life emergency up on the roof, she hurried the children back to class. I was told later that one of the man's own children was in that class.

We had been at it for about twenty-five minutes when I turned to the rest of the team and said, "He's had no heart-beat, no spontaneous respirations for a long time now. I don't think we're going to get anywhere. I think we should call it. I don't know what we're accomplishing." The ER docs agreed and we stopped. It is a terrible moment when you finally stop a resuscitation. There are no rules about what happens then. One minute you are directing every possible thought and action to saving someone, the next minute, nothing—nothing but an odd-shaped void in which every word and every move seems wrong. It feels like gears grinding, screeching inside. It is a moment full of losing, and pain and tears are only inches away. We covered the man with a sheet and then stepped back. I couldn't look up at our audience. Impossible as the odds had been, I was overwhelmed by the very public nature of the defeat. I wondered what all those patients were think-ing as they walked away from their windows. I wondered if death felt a little closer, a little more inevitable than ever. For the first time I noticed my shirt, the mop bucket in the corner, the coldness in the shadow. I began to shake, uncontrollably.

"We'll take it from here, Dr. Judge," someone said. The head nurse and I walked over to the edge of the roof and backed down the long ladder to the pavement below.

"You'd better change your shirt, Jim," Sherri whispered as we stood on the driveway.

I was numb. I walked down the hall to the surgical locker room, took off my shirt and undershirt, and threw them both away. I put on a scrub top and walked back out into the hall. One of the administrators stopped me and said the police were there and that they needed to question me and the medical students, since we were the primary eyewitnesses.

I sat in the administrator's office and ran through the story, clutching a cup of coffee someone had handed me. I think I held it more for warmth than anything else. I didn't even drink coffee. Step by step, I told the officers what had happened. They were businesslike and acted as if this was all pretty routine. They wanted to be convinced that there was no foul play. I remember them asking if I was sure there was no one else in the room with him at the time he jumped. I hesitated before answering. I just didn't want to believe anyone could have done that on their own.

Over the next two days the hospital grapevine provided a lot more detail to the man's story. I was right about seeing him in the postop area, but that had been several months before. He had initially worked as a nurse's aide. He had served as a medic in Vietnam and was pursuing some kind of further training. He had a wife and two children and no big problems he had ever talked to anyone about, but it wasn't long before things started to unravel. He began to withdraw from friends and family, eventually into a shell not even his wife could penetrate. Over the months, his performance at work took a parallel downhill course. The nursing supervisor, trying to be protective, had gradually put him into roles of less and less responsibility. But soon it was apparent that any patient-care role was not appropriate. She had talked to the director of maintenance and was able to get him transferred so at least he could stay employed. His detachment only progressed. Recently he had started meeting with personnel, who urged him to get some counseling. No one knew whether he had or not. Over the last several weeks, many people reported seeing him standing in the hallway at night, for long stretches of time, holding on to his mop, just staring into the dark.

By putting together the statements of more than twenty witnesses, a clearer picture of the morning of the jump came into focus. At least forty people had passed by him in the service room that morning. Some said they spoke; most did not. None of them got any response from him. His supervisor had tried several times to locate him but the man at the window had stepped into a world beyond the range of any pager. Maybe inside he was doing some kind of final battle with the dragons of his past that were slowly consuming him. We could all guess at what they might have been. Maybe it was something unimaginable that he had brought back from Vietnam, some terrible memory lodged deep down inside. Maybe it was the unbearable pain of the world in which he was now trapped; a world that not only didn't understand, but didn't even want to hear about it. Whatever it was, he struggled with it alone, not noticing and for the most part going unnoticed by the world around him. It was determined that he had been standing in the same position, staring out that window, for almost two hours before he jumped.

I was a semicelebrity around the hospital for the next couple of weeks. The eyewitness doctor who saw the guy jump, ran down five flights of stairs, "got all tore up" getting out onto the roof, then tried to save him. I had been quoted in the papers, and it seemed everyone wanted to talk to me. The problem was that I didn't feel very heroic. I was traumatized for weeks afterward but I never told anyone. I guess I thought heroes were supposed to be strong and just move on to the next fight. "Get a grip; put it behind you; be strong," blared like propaganda in my head. But I felt a strong countercurrent churning just below the surface, and at times it felt like I was in danger of being swept away. I was jumpy. Every loud noise startled me, and each time it happened I heard the crashing of glass all over again. I was haunted with flashbacks, especially of that one moment when he looked straight into my eyes just before leaping to his death. I am sure the actual length of that moment was no more than a heartbeat, but rerunning it so many times had made it feature-length. Like two people sitting at their respective windows in trains running fast down parallel tracks, for a moment we were traveling together, then one of us lurched forward. I could have sworn that as we connected in that final moment, there were unmouthed words that passed between us. But the words were in a language I didn't speak. I've never been quite sure whether the last look of the man at the window said, "Please, give me a reason not to do this," or "Please don't."

I had faced more gruesome things in my career so far, but none affected me the way this did. I kept asking myself why. Part of it was how meaningless it all felt. I couldn't shake the thought that mine was the last face he saw and he saw nothing there to hold him back. Why did it have to happen at all?

I drifted back to his isolation, to his slow, gradual withdrawal from this world into the dark world of his own making. He had disconnected and paid the price. The more I thought about it, the more this man's suicide made the absurdity of treating people without really taking the time to know them all the more acute. Could anything have held him back that morning, if only for a moment—a moment long enough to get to that room and stop him? If anything could have, I was sure it had little to do with a white coat or a medical degree. Maybe a human touch, some reason to hope. Some connection. Then again, maybe he had traveled past the human frontier to a place beyond the reach of human hands. Maybe he was convinced only God could free him, and he knew of no other way to get to him. When he leaped out of that window that morning, I wondered, did he think he would fall or fly?

It took months for the flashbacks to stop, months to stop jumping every time there was a loud noise. Months to be able to walk past that service room on the eighth floor without stopping to stare and rerun the whole tape. Months to be able to look out a window at the hospital and not have my gaze drawn to all the other windows, wondering how many others stood at those windows fighting the same kind of battle. Months passed and it all slowly faded. Yet I found that in the end, time did not bring me as much healing as it did burial. Eventually, the memories and emotions were buried by the daily stuff of life that so often crowds out true living. Bills to pay, patients to see, a family to take care of, a future to plan. Even the flashbacks of that final moment began to dim. But before they did, one chilling aspect changed—whenever I relived that last moment, when I looked into his face right before he jumped, it was no longer his face staring back at me.

It was my own.

POSTSCRIPT

I never heard anything further about what happened to the man's family. There was some talk about his wife threatening to sue the hospital, but that never materialized. I thought about trying to find her and tell her about the last minutes of his life, but the more I thought about it the more it seemed that anything I had to say would only compound her pain. For years afterward, I could barely keep my emotions under control whenever I recounted the story. Why? What was still so unresolved? I think more than anything else, this incident forced me to face my own fear of the dark. Not the physical dark, but the spiritual dark—the dark reality that a person could actually come to a place where there was no hope left. I was frightened by the depth of this man's darkness. How did he arrive at a place where only death offered a modicum of hope? Did he plunge headlong into that darkness, or did whatever light he had in his life just slowly fade away? How many times had God offered him a lifeline, a candle, something to bring him back? There were so many people surrounding him, and yet he saw no one. And that morning of his death, as he gazed out the window at that beautiful blue sky, was he really just plotting an escape or was he searching, no matter how misguidedly, for a doorway to heaven? I couldn't help wondering how many other people, desperate and with very little hope left, shared elevators with me, sat beside me in cafeterias, walked by me in hallways. Or maybe even spoke to me from hospital beds, spoke about everything except what was really hurting them. Afraid to say it. Maybe hiding behind a childlike last hope that if the question is yet to be asked, there still remains at least the possibility of an answer.

I made myself a promise. I would look for them. I would ask the probing and important questions, the ones that had nothing to do with their illness and everything to do with it at the same time. I would search the faces of the people who crossed my path for any trace of resemblance to the man at the window. There would be one person in this world that would be able to say that his death was not without meaning.

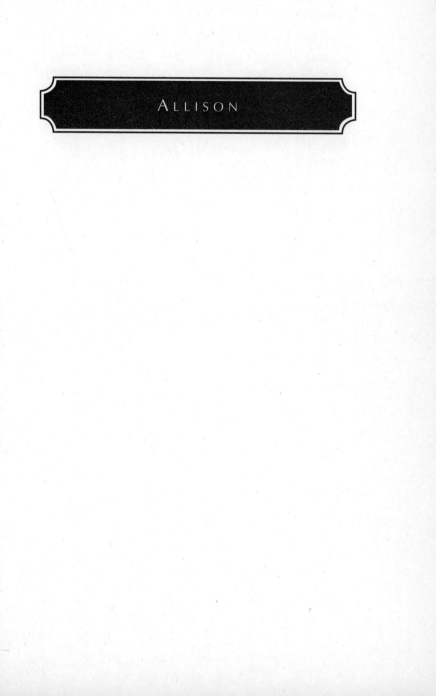

ALLISON

She sat there smiling, her hands gripping the sides of the exam table, rocking back and forth. Her shoulders were hunched slightly forward, and she looked almost like a five-year-old on a rocking chair designed for someone much more grown up. Her head was tilted just to one side, and her fine golden-streaked hair swung forward with each rocking motion. As if describing having been caught sneaking cookies, she began her story.

"I know, I know. We should have waited, but we just couldn't." Smile. "Anyway, we're going to get married in a few months, so I guess it doesn't really matter that much. I don't know what my parents are so upset about. I don't think it's really a big deal. So what if we're a little young. We were going to get married when Tom got out of the army in two years, so . . . now we'll just get married sooner." Smile.

Listening to her, I was struck by two things. First, she was going way beyond what I would describe as "putting a good spin on things." She was eighteen, pregnant, unmarried, and barely out of high school. Yet the danger or the risk or the sadness or the lost opportunities or the just plain "not ready yet" of her teenage pregnancy were not allowed anywhere near. As soon as anything negative approached, she would wave it away like so much smoke drifting her way from a campfire. I was impressed by the fact that I seemed to be pretty superfluous to this conversation. She was talking too fast and with a kind of urgency I often see in patients when the person they are most trying to convince is themselves. I had a very deep sense I was listening to something she had already rehearsed a hundred times over in the morning-mirror of her mind.

She was in my office that day to begin prenatal care. I didn't know Ali all that well. I think I had only seen her once or twice before, mostly for sore throats and such. We completed her initial physical exam that morning, and everything seemed normal enough. The baby's size and the date of conception were consistent with one another. Her routine blood work was all normal. Her monologue continued.

"I'm sorry you won't get to deliver the baby. I hope you don't mind, but see, I'm leaving for Germany in July. Tom and I have decided to get married over there, and then I'll just deliver the baby in the army hospital there. Tom's looking for an apartment for us right now. We already talked it over and I don't want to live on the base. That will be kinda cool won't it, having the baby born in another country? The doctors at the base are all Americans."

I had only been in practice about three years, and this instant intimacy that characterized my visits with patients still felt strange. The scene usually played out like this: The door to the examination room would close and I could see the patient's search begin, their thoughts almost readable. *Is this someone I can trust, someone who cares?* And when the answer to that question came back *Yes,* the sliding panel on the confessional was thrown back and the sacrament began. Patients I had seen at most once or twice would, with startling regularity, lay bare their entire lives; tell me things that their priests and pastors and even spouses had never heard, would never hear. Then the second stage of the search would begin as they searched my face for traces of judgment or rejection or understanding or absolution—maybe absolution most of all. I was developing the art of medicine, and part of that art is the ability to listen to the most horrendous details without allowing what's going on inside to find any translation on your face.

I was definitely working at keeping what was going on inside me from finding its way out that morning with Ali. As I heard her describe in great detail how her life was going to all work out, what I was thinking was that this package was wrapped just a little too neatly. Her carefully constructed script was just this side of a romance novel. It had everything—passion, impetuous lovers, disapproving family, a move to a new world where the new little family, complete with bundle of joy, would begin life happily. It had everything except the white picket fence and the rosebushes. I studied her as she went on. There was something about Ali that made you want to protect her. I don't know exactly what it was. Maybe it was her childlike manner, or the almost sparkling innocence that made you forgive her naiveté. Maybe it was the insidious feeling that not even she believed what she was saying. Inside, my cynical side was doing battle with that other part in which hope hides out. Deep down I wanted her happily-ever-after to happen for her. I wanted her to be the winner of the life lotto, to be that one person for whom it all does go according to plan. I wanted her script, someone's script, to run without edit. But just when the hope inside started taking hold a shadow fell across the scene, a shadow cast by hard reality. And my own internal dialogue began.

Come on, get a grip, I thought. *The father of this baby is hardly a shining model of responsibility. Since when did getting a girl pregnant initiate a life-changing "coming to your senses" for the average nineteen-year-old male in America?* I shook it off.

"Well, however it all works out, your health and the baby's health are our first priorities here." And I proceeded to give my happy Dr. Judge prenatal instructions, tape number 101, about the importance of diet and exercise and prenatal vitamins and what to avoid and what to get plenty of and everything else that at this one moment did not matter because she wanted, she needed, something else from me right then. I could tell by the look on her face. She wanted something real, some affirmation that the future she had just prophesied for herself was more than a pretty fantasy. But I couldn't give it to her and carefully avoided the question.

We did the same dance at some point during most of our monthly visits. She was looking ahead to her trip to Germany, the details of which she went on and on and on about. More details than I needed, certainly, and yet I couldn't quite extinguish that part of me that wanted to cheer her on. Her voice continued to have that need to convince mixed with excitement. She had a demeanor you often see in a group of adolescent girls fidgeting in line for the big roller coaster, trying to convince themselves that at the last minute they won't chicken out. I found her anticipation contagious, and at times I forgot my own doubts and joined in.

Her last visit before leaving for Germany finally came. We talked over the details of getting all her records transferred and made sure she understood her future visit schedule. She hugged me, and I responded awkwardly, as always, said good-bye, and watched her leave the office into a future I hoped would be good.

I thought of her often over the next month, wondering how it was all going. I got a definitive answer six weeks later. I was surprised to see her name on my schedule one morning. The moment I opened the exam room door I knew instantly that something had gone very wrong. Ali had run headlong into an oncoming train called reality, and she had come out on the bad side of the collision. The person I saw sitting on the exam table was not remotely the same bubbly person I had seen in the previous months. She was dull, spoke slowly, and the spark of life that had been so characteristic of her before was absent.

She told a story that went beyond even my most pessimistic predictions. Her reception in Germany by the baby's father had been anything but warm. Apparently, he had not been all that serious about her coming over, and the first thing he did was express surprise that Ali intended to stay. He talked awkwardly about what his life was like in the army, emphasizing how much he liked it, how much partying he did, the guys in his barracks, and each of their peculiarities. Ali excused this all in her head and told herself that it was all part of getting used to one another again and that he'd relax in a few days.

The second day they were together went worse. One of the first questions he had that morning was about the possibility of adoption, and it quickly deteriorated from there. Not even Allison's perpetual optimism could recast the events or his attitude. He was a soldier, and there was no room in his life for a wife and baby right now. It became obvious, even to Ali, that he had no intention of marrying her and didn't want any involvement with the baby. "Why didn't you just get an abortion when there was still time?" was the question that sliced particularly deep. She returned home emotionally cut and was still bleeding.

"It's his baby too," she muttered, shaking her head, speaking slowly, carefully. There was very little eye contact, and I knew I was only a surrogate in this conversation, a stand-in for someone else. Maybe the real dialogue was with herself, or her boyfriend. Maybe it was with God. I couldn't shake thinking that if I had said anything even halfway insightful or penetrating or wise, she would have looked up, surprised to see me there. "How could he talk about giving it away or killing it?" she went on. I think the real question thundering in her head was a simpler one: How could he not care? That question's volume drowned out the sound of almost everything else. I think she desperately wanted an answer, yet she feared what that answer might be. I believe it was the most serious question of her life till then. How could he not care?

Eighty percent of those who see a family doctor are women, and over time one gets to listen to many real-life examples of how, as a gender, men can leave a lot to be desired. You would think I would have had enough experience to be accustomed to the stories in which the basic theme is, "All men are idiots." But hearing the stories of male dereliction always causes a mixed emotional soup to stew inside me. On the one hand it makes me feel shame for my gender, and I find myself compelled to try to convince the person I am listening to that not all men are complete jerks. (Although for the life of me, I consistently have trouble coming up with an example of someone who isn't.) On the other hand, there is a certain element of vicarious guilt that results from the knowledge that if I were really truthful, I would have to say that the accusation, whatever it is, probably fits me as well. In Ali's case, I stayed silent and did what men do best in awkward situations—changed the subject. I drew the focus instead toward the one undeniably good thing about this whole situation: the baby.

Allison continued to vent at all her subsequent prenatal visits; but her speech was mostly mutterings, abbreviated and coded reports from the emotional fronts upon which she was doing battle that week. Her parents . . . she was living at home. Her dad was mostly silent, but his silence was a weapon that, in some ways, wounded more than any words could have. Her mom tried to be supportive, but there were comments she couldn't keep to herself. Comments into which Ali read messages of shame and accusation and "I told you so," and it was these that Ali held on to. But neither her father's withdrawal nor her mothers outbursts came close to the hostility she saw looking back at herself in the mirror. No one's derision was more relentless than her own. She felt stupid, taken in, used, and discarded. She felt duped, not just by her boyfriend, but by a set of assumptions about life that now seemed so juvenile. It was as if she had spent her whole life believing the world was one way and then, in one shocking moment, had learned that everything she believed in, everything she had counted on, was fiction. We didn't talk much about God, although we should have, because that was probably the assumption she wrestled with most. As her world came crashing in I think it was her view of God that was challenged most. Wasn't he supposed to be the benevolent old grandfather that pats you on the head and finds something good to say about you even when you're at your worst? A kindly old gentleman who, either by choice or absentmindedness, looks the other way when it comes to his grandchildren's faults and failures? Who, no matter what else is going on, always has a piece of candy ready in his pocket?

Ali was experiencing the death of a dream, maybe a lot of dreams all at once. What she needed most from me at that point was comfort, but I was pretty new at all of this, and "comfort" is not a class you take in medical school. Like most heart skills, it comes only with practice, and I was still very much in the learning process on that one. Often, I think, what patients long for, maybe what we all long for most deeply, is simply the knowledge that they are not alone; that there is one other human being who has heard the whole story, has listened, and cares. Many times, doctors are called on to be not so much scientists as storytellers. Whether it is cancer or a cold, patients simply want someone to say, "I know of others who have traveled this same road and have gotten through, maybe not always to their stated destination but at least to a destination that turned out all right." The value of that, the life it imparts, and the high cost of delivering it in this world are all grossly underestimated.

And so I practiced the ancient art of comfort on Allison, not knowing then just how much practice she would give me. I am sure, looking back now, that I stumbled significantly, but I think she was able to forgive my clumsiness and accept my intent, even if the substance of my comfort was at times somewhat lacking. And in the process, we became friends.

It was two weeks before her due date, and she came in for a routine check. She spontaneously said, "Well, I think I am going to be early. I haven't felt the baby move much lately, and my mother said that's sometimes a sign that labor is going to start soon."

I laughed and said there is not much that happens to a woman in the last month of her pregnancy that is not a sign that labor's about to begin according to somebody's science. What I was really thinking was that a change in the baby's movement pattern can mean a lot of things, most of them not good. But I tried not to let on as I placed the Doppler scope on her abdomen to listen to the baby's heart tones. Silence. I checked the scope to make sure it was functioning and tried in several different places, pressing a little harder each time, but in each place I got the same result. Nothing, nothing at all, and I felt myself go pale. A fetal demise—the baby was dead, I was sure of it. I began to stagger under the crushing weight of that knowledge.

"Allison, I'm having a hard time hearing the baby right now. Sometimes that simply means that the baby is in a position where the heartbeat is obscured, covered over by the mother's heartbeat, but I think just to be safe I'm going to send you down the hall to the ultrasound and just confirm that everything is all right." I knew when I sent her down that hallway that there was a high likelihood they would confirm an intrauterine death. My heart was in my throat as I called the ultrasound tech and warned her of my suspicions. I watched Allison walk slowly down the hallway, then she turned back, the look on her face begging me not to let this happen. I stood powerless and tried to smile a reassuring smile, knowing that my face was not conforming to the lie.

As she disappeared around the corner, I felt something happen inside. It is, I believe, a common occurrence with doctors, although I've never actually talked about it with my colleagues. When a patient experiences a "bad result," a bad diagnosis or a complication of some type, a toxic brew begins to bubble up inside—panic and fear and guilt and failure. It has a remarkably heavy sense of déjà vu, like when I was a medical student and couldn't answer the arrogant chief resident's impossible questions. Only this time the exam's for real. You can try denial for a while, but you soon find it's a flimsy stronghold. Even though the math is with you—the vast majority of patients do get better—you can't delude yourself forever into thinking that everyone gets better and there's always a cure and everyone comes back and thanks you. At this moment I found myself clinging irrationally to this hope, denying the dark reality that eventually the numbers catch up with you. And when it's not true, when the tragedy occurs, and people don't get better, and there is no cure, it doesn't matter how unequivocally the facts point out that it wasn't your fault. The truth is, something terrible happened on your watch, and there is a certain guilt by association that begins to seep through the walls of your straw fortress.

Ten minutes later the ultrasound tech called me out of a room. I was right. The baby was dead. A couple of days at least. The ultrasound showed the classic signs of an intra-uterine death. No heart activity, the child's eggshell-like skull bones overriding one another. I asked the tech to bring Allison back into a room.

Without anyone saying anything, I believe she already knew, but the words needed to be said. They would be the handle by which we could both begin to grasp the tragedy of all this. "Ali, something terrible has happened. We don't know why, but your baby has died inside you." Ali broke down sobbing. I paused, swallowed, and gave her some time, although an eternity of time would not have answered the questions pounding inside her right then. With tragic news, there is both a how and a why that must be answered in some way before any patient can begin to experience healing and move on. The doctor can often answer the how, but the why belongs to God and is almost never quickly answered.

I stood silently, watching her, feeling that the painful intimacy of this moment was a holy thing I had no right to look upon. I was just quiet and fought back my own emotions, though why I felt that was so important to do right then I still don't know. What I wanted to do, what I felt an overwhelming urge to do, was to put my arm around her and cry with her for this baby and for her and for me and for this poor sad world where pain is so often on parade. I could almost see her sag beneath the overwhelming weight of guilt and judgment. I wanted to relieve it in some way, but absolution is never ours to give; it is the gift of God. I wanted to say that this tragedy has nothing to do with judgment. What's happened here is lousy but it just happens sometimes. People get sick and die and bad things happen and that is just the way it is. I wish it wasn't happening to you and I hope it never happens to me but the whole point is that it has and it will, and if I could be a real human being right now I would tell you that it scares me too. But you are not being singled out, your crimes are no worse than mine. I wanted to tell her that what she was feeling inside could not possibly be coming from God, that it was coming from the dark reaches of her own heart. I wanted to plead with her not to listen to that voice.

But I said none of this. Instead, I waited for a moment of control to come and then, putting on my professional armor, I explained the facts of what needed to happen next. I spoke slowly and deliberately. As much for my benefit as for hers.

"Ali, the ultrasound looks as if the baby has been dead for several days. This can be a dangerous thing for the mother, so it's important that the baby be delivered as soon as possible." I searched for the right thing to say. Words like mother and baby and birth felt hollow and wrong, but I could find no others to take their place.

I've found that patients look to hear only certain things from certain people. From the doctor they look for a basic message. "You are okay, the shadow on the x-ray is nothing, or it's something but there is a treatment." The doctor delivers the big news. The details are best delivered by someone else. It's as if the patient visualizes you, the physician, over and over again saying the same thing and won't let other words come out.

"I'm going to meet you over at the hospital in a couple of hours. My nurse is going to come in right now and explain where you need to go and what happens from here. Should we call your parents to come pick you up?" This last question yanked her back from wherever she was at that moment, and startled she said, "No, no that's okay, I'm okay. I'll go home and tell them." The intensity of her response made me wonder what waited for her at home. Would it be the judgment she felt or the compassion she needed?

I finished that day's patients, called my wife to explain that I would be at the hospital for most of the evening, then headed to the labor and delivery suite. When I arrived I could tell the nurses were working at not having to be the one to take care of my patient, and that was understandable. Death was certainly not the reason they went into obstetrical nursing. A very compassionate newer graduate got the short straw. She had never had a child herself, and that may have made it a little easier for her than for the others. Ali arrived, and I went into her room and explained what was about to happen, about the Pitocin to stimulate labor and the monitor to measure the contractions' strength. Ali was mostly blank, stoic, on merciful autopilot, resigning herself in whatever way she could to what was coming.

I sat in the doctors' lounge waiting, and as I waited I pushed away the real conversation that labored inside me— the one that pressured me to ask myself some of the same dangerous questions with which Ali must have struggled. Dangerous questions that carry the risk of experiencing the patient's pain by proxy. I was already relatively skilled at pretend-and-avoid maneuvers and was actively engaged in both. Pretending came first. I pretended that what I was caught up in was nothing more than patient and doctor. Clean and simple. I was here to render a medical service . . . that was it. But I couldn't pretend away the reality that beyond patient and doctor we were two fellow human beings, sharing the same space, breathing the same air, feeling many of the same feelings, fearing the same monsters under the bed. Probably crying out right now to the same Father. As the hours dragged on and pretending broke down, I turned to avoidance, another old friend. I used a trick I'd learned indirectly in medical school: fill up on facts and maybe there won't be any room left for feelings. I sat there in that room for hours and pored over several ancient issues of *Time* magazine, reading voraciously about things that didn't interest me in the least. It was volume I was looking for, hoping that the sheer volume of information might push away the feelings. CNN blah, blah, blahed in the corner of the room. Farm commodity prices and weather patterns and inscrutable foreign policy issues became the blankets under which I sought refuge—refuge from the suspicion that although God is always with you in the dark, it's his fingerprints on the light switch.

This was how I waited for my moment upon the stage of the drama playing itself out down the hall. I checked in on Ali several times over the next few hours, but as much as I tried, I couldn't break through the protective shell she had built around herself. It was an out-of-sync experience for me. I had delivered another baby in this same delivery room, at almost the same time, with the same nurse the day before. That was a perfect delivery. A loving dad, a stable home, a second child, this time a girl. Everything had gone as if scripted to perfection. Now, we were in a different universe.

In the early morning hours, the call from the nurse finally came. "I think we're ready for you." I took a deep breath and walked down the hall to Ali's room and quickly checked her. She was fully dilated, and the baby's head was beginning its descent down the birth canal. The nurse and I talked to Ali about pushing. Everything was in slow motion, as if we were walking through a dress rehearsal instead of the real thing. I was surprised that Ali's mother was not in the delivery room with us, but I was pretty sure that had been Ali's decision. She did not want anyone else in the room with her—I think she didn't even want us there. So her parents sat by themselves outside the labor area, waiting. Ali had chosen to take this road alone. Throughout the entire labor and delivery she remained quiet and almost detached, avoiding eye contact whenever she could. She smiled politely. I think detaching from it all was the only way she had of making it through.

As the baby's head began to appear, I detected the un-mistakable feel of the overriding skull bones, which took away even that small hope of the hopeless that seems to remain until the inevitable actually happens. The umbilical cord was wrapped in a tight noose around the child's neck, the most likely answer to how the child had died, and I had to cut it before delivering the rest of the baby. With one final push, all of the baby was delivered. A tiny limp and lifeless little girl. I handed the baby to the nurse, who wrapped the baby in a small pink blanket and placed a tiny stocking cap over her misshapen head. She glanced over at me, her tear-filled eyes flashing above her mask, asking without words whether she should give the baby to Ali. I nodded, and as Ali reached up and cradled her baby, she began for the first time to gently cry as she brushed the baby's hair with her hand and touched her tiny fingers. I was thankful that I had a mask to hide behind and the remainder of the delivery to attend to. The placenta and the stitches and the instruments and the routine were for me a grace and mercy all their own.

Ali's muffled crying continued. I finished what needed to be done, then stepped over to the head of the bed. A single surgical light shining down from the ceiling lighted the room and created an almost surreal setting, like a black-and-white drama. I felt myself shuddering inside as I took in the whole scene: the baby's putty-gray color, Ali's quiet sobs, and my own emptiness in the face of it all. I mumbled through some postdelivery instructions and then after a moment of silence, knowing Ali had not heard a word of what I just said, did maybe the one truly spontaneous, human thing I managed to do that evening. I reached forward, gently touching the child's cheek with my finger and said, "She was such a pretty little thing."

I fought for control as Ali and I connected for a moment and the line between patient and doctor blurred. I walked over to the side of the room and began to write postpartum orders. Then I went to the locker room, changed clothes, and walked down the long and empty hallways to the lot where I had parked my car. I opened the door, got behind the wheel, and as I fumbled with the keys at the ignition suddenly broke down crying, sobbing like a child who just doesn't care or like a mother who cares too much. I cried for the baby and for Ali and for me having to be a part of it. The faces of my own three daughters, all younger than five, flashed in front of me, and I was overwhelmed with the heavy reminder that they could be taken away from me some day in some way just as random and reasonless. It slapped me in the face and I sat there stinging from it. I think there were also tears of frustration and a little shame—the shame of hiding my own tears, of not being human enough to share in Ali's grief, of hiding behind the image of an in-control physician. I reasoned that it was really what she had needed at that moment. I knew it was an excuse.

I arrived home at about 2:00 A.M. My wife turned toward me and sleepily asked how everything went. I simply said it went as well as could be expected, rolled over, and fell asleep, telling myself I would tell her later what it had been like and how ashamed I felt and how frightened it had made me. Yes, that was right, I would tell her all about it. Maybe the next morning. I fell asleep rehearsing what I would say.

But I never did.

POSTSCRIPT

Ali continued to live with her parents, and I think they grew into a new relationship in the shadow of her tragedy. She did find a level of comfort in them. She went to the junior college nearby and eventually got a good job. There was a guardedness that became a part of her, a kind of growing up. In some ways I missed that naive girl she had been, the one who saw only good things for her future. She married about five years later, a quiet guy. They had two sons. Shortly after the birth of her second son they moved out of state. She sent me a card telling me they had just bought their first home, thanking me for being her doctor. I smiled when I got the note, pretty sure the new house must have a white picket fence and some rosebushes.

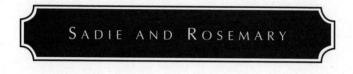

SADIE AND ROSEMARY

One of the things my training definitely failed to prepare me for was how often I would have to work at not laughing. I guess that's understandable. If surprise is the key element of humor, a doctor's office certainly provides lots of opportunity for that. As my practice developed, it amazed me how many times in a day I had to keep the smile under wraps. Although "a merry heart doeth good like medicine," I have learned that if you don't use it with caution, you're not likely to strengthen the patient-doctor relationship—particularly when it's the patient generating the smiles.

Something strange happens when the door to the exam room closes. It's apparently all some patients need to suddenly feel free and let it all loose. I don't fully appreciate the dynamic. Maybe when patients find themselves alone with you in the exam room it occurs to them, *Hey, I've got a captive audience!* It must seem like a safe place to let down, be themselves, and see if something they've been thinking about or doing is really that crazy or not. Whenever I speak with colleagues who find nothing funny in their daily practices, I can only think that either they just aren't paying attention or they have lost something essential to surviving in private practice—a sense of humor.

For some reason, many of my more humorous encounters have come through the lives of older female patients. I think, as a group, these ladies have spent much of their lives strapped into the tight girdle of "propriety"; holding things in, sure that by doing so they are keeping the very fabric of civilization from unraveling. Who knows, maybe they're right. But as the finish line comes into sight, so to speak, I have observed that they often adopt new attitudes and behaviors that must feel pretty darned good. There were two older ladies I cared for at about the same time that were good examples of this phenomenon. They both lived in worlds that, over the years, were more and more of their own making, worlds into which I made regular house calls.

The first was named Sadie and she was in her mid seventies. She was a great ocean liner of a lady who cut a wide berth as she cruised down the hall with her walker. My nurse on one side and her husband on the other served as tugboats, bumping her gently back into the main channel of the hallway. Sadie always looked as if someone had just grabbed a stocking cap off her head. Her hair was so full of static electricity that I always thought twice before placing a stethoscope on her, half afraid I'd initiate an arc of lightning and blow us both into the next county. She was in the very earliest stages of dementia or senility, and one of the first things she taught me was that, at least in its early stages, not being "all there" comes with a few perks. It affords one the opportunity to be excused for just about any outrageous behavior one might come up with. As I got to know her better, I became less and less sure as to how many of Sadie's shenanigans were induced by the foreknowledge that she would be easily forgiven. These suspicions were only compounded by Sadie's nearly constant "cat that swallowed the canary" smile.

I really liked Sadie. No matter how outrageous or blunt she might be, you just couldn't help but like her. She was the quintessential wacky grandmother, the one grandchildren tell stories about for the next fifty years. She was completely unpredictable. Sometimes she would show up at visits with two purses or her sweater on inside out. There was no subject off-limits for her, and because of how slowly she moved down the hall and how loudly she spoke, everyone in the clinic got an earful. Her complete freedom to just say whatever she liked was a big part of why I always looked forward to seeing her name on my schedule.

Her husband, Frank, was there faithfully at each and every visit. I think it was his idea to switch doctors and start seeing me in the first place, probably in the hope that a fresh face might generate some improvement in his wife's chronic medical condition. Frank was an ex-marine, a big old billy goat of a character with gruff and salty language. He always wore the same cap and the same brown high-water double-knit slacks, hiked like Tweedledee, about five inches above his true waist. But in sharp contrast to his general demeanor, Frank feigned over his wife like an insecure courtier, never quite sure whether he was in or out of favor. I hate to say it, but I think it was exactly where Sadie wanted him. I have generally observed this kind of behavior in men either looking hard for a purpose in life or working out some kind of penance. If Frank was guilty, I thankfully never determined the exact nature of his sins. Whatever his reason, he treated Sadie like a porcelain doll. Now well into retirement, Sadie had become his full-time job, and maybe they were both the better for it. Frank had something to do, and Sadie was getting the full focus, controlling the show, perhaps for the first time in their entire marriage. There was an odd justice to it all.

Sadie had all the problems that accompany living seventy-plus years on the planet—severe arthritis, frequent bladder infections, decreased hearing, congestive heart failure, and now the beginnings of dementia. Age had thinned the filter most of us use in our daily interactions with others, leaving Sadie pretty free to tell you exactly how she felt about things. And she did, in a heavy Polish accent.

"Them new blue pills you give me, Dr. Judge, I gotta tell ya, dey just don't do one blasted thing for me. Now old Dr. Newton used to give me the B_{12} shots and, ohhhhh, did they ever give me da energy. I'm telling you. Why don't you give me doze shots?"

Dr. Newton, who had retired fifteen years before at the age of eighty-five, was legendary with patients and doctors alike. For different reasons, of course. Just about every doctor in town had some of his old patients in their practice and we all had suffered through the testimonials of how much better they all felt with his injections. The doctors, however, knew something the patients did not. Those "B_{12}" injections often had a little bit more than B_{12} in them. Dr. Newton's shots contained everything from thyroid hormone to cortisone to extracted horse gonads.

"Now, Sadie, you know we don't use those injections anymore," I replied. I had learned early in my relationship with Sadie that complex medical explanations were not what she was usually looking for. Keep it simple. What Sadie needed more than anything else was some basic handholding. Although most of our visits consisted of mild adjustments to an already finely tuned medical regimen, the real therapy, and maybe the real purpose of those visits, was so Sadie could tell her story and be listened to and simply be touched. Many studies have shown that for a majority of older patients, the doctor's office is the only place where they are actually physically touched by another human being. And there, I think, lay the real value of our visits, because heaven knows there was nothing much else likely to improve her deteriorating medical condition. Somehow she felt better after each visit, and she would always grab my hand and squeeze it hard and thank me profusely. She taught me the therapeutic value of just listening, and she returned like clockwork, the first Monday of every month, for more.

There was one particularly memorable Monday. My schedule simply read: "Sadie A.—Check personal problem."

Now, doctors learn to dread any patient encounter that has "personal" as the reason for the appointment, because that is almost never good news. You can generally guess at what it means depending on the patient's age and sex. If it's a teenage girl, most likely, she is coming in to talk about birth control. If it's a woman between thirty and fifty, it's more than likely her marriage or depression. And if it's a man, no matter what the age, bet on it being worries regarding something going wrong just south of his beltline, and he didn't want to explain it to the person making the appointment. But as I looked at my schedule I couldn't predict what it meant for a seventy-year-old woman. The truth was, I could never have guessed what concerned Sadie that day. I sat down in the exam room across from Sadie. Frank, as usual, was standing just behind her, looking grimmer than he normally did. There was a long period of silence while she gave me her Cheshire grin, which always seemed to indicate the two of us had some kind of secret, a secret she never let me in on.

She looked at me and then in her truly unique voice—a blend of Edith Bunker with Daffy Duck—she said, "Dr. Judge, I know people. I know dey talk, but I just want you to know something . . . I am not a prostitute."

Whoaaaa, hold the phone. Somebody's reality check just bounced. I sat there with my empathetic Dr. Judge smile frozen on my face, just blinking, my thoughts racing. *What did she say?* I was sure I had not heard her correctly. Of all the words that could have ended that sentence, *prostitute* was not on the option list. *Protestant, protester, proselytizer, prostate* might even have been accepted as a correct answer, but not *prostitute*.

So, walking right into it, I shook my head and said, "I'm sorry, Sadie, what did you say?"

She grabbed my hand and with the utmost sincerity, her sad brown eyes imploring me not to believe it, said, "I'm not, Dr. Judge, I am not a prostitute. I know da people talk, I heard them, and I want you to know da truth."

I groped for my next line. What was I supposed to say? Was I supposed to say what I was really thinking right then? Because what I was thinking was that if I had made a short list of all the people in the world I was pretty sure were not prostitutes, Sadie would have definitely ranked in the top five, along with Mother Teresa and my mom.

I turned to her husband, searching for some kind of help, but he just stood there shaking his head. Then in a short scrappy voice, as if he couldn't take the shame of it, he said, "I never heard 'em say it, but if I did I'd, I'd . . . why I'd knock it out of 'em!"

Ooooooookay, I thought looking from him to her, then back again. *Obviously no help coming from that direction.*

Time to regroup.

I struggled with what to do at this point. Do I . . .

1. assume they are victims of a group delusion and shoot for family therapy,

2. try to gently ease her out of it from the inside, play into the situation, or

3. maybe just change the subject and start talking about the weather?

I chose door #2, took a deep breath, and jumped right in. I assured Sadie that she must not have heard properly and that no one would ever say that about her, and even if they did I certainly would never believe it. (As I said it I suddenly realized that there I was, sucked right into the delusion with them!) I moved quickly to the rest of her exam, making a mental note to check her old records to see when she had last had her hearing checked.

When Sadie left that morning she did as she always did, patted me on the hand, thanked me for helping her, told me how much better she felt, and cruised toward reception. She paused her walker at the end of the hallway, turned, and gave me that same old grin, this time with a little wink. To this day I still don't know if she was serious or not.

At about the same time another older lady arrived in my life whose name was Rosemary.

Whereas Sadie, with all her quirks, was almost instantly likable, Rosemary's initial impact on me was very different. She was only in her mid sixties, but she looked and acted a good deal older. Her hair was a perfect halo of mouse-brown duck fluff that seemed to have a life of its own. At a little over 200 pounds and a little under five feet tall the word that seemed to describe her best was simply "round." She had an irritated expression on her face that almost never changed. If you saw her on the street, you would automatically classify her as a grumpy little old lady. Over time I learned that Rosemary lived in a perpetual state of estrangement. She was on the outs with her children, her pastor, her hairdresser, her newspaper boy, and most of the doctors who had ever seen her. She had the gift of being contrary and felt compelled to tell everyone, no matter what they said, why what they had said was not entirely correct. Over time my encounters with Rosemary became the experiential equivalent of fingernails on the chalkboard.

Rosemary had made a small cottage industry out of her perceived medical needs, and I was just one doctor in a long list of MDs, DOs, chiropractors, ophthalmologists, and podiatrists who, according to Rosemary, vacillated between saving her from some dreaded fate and doing her in. Rosemary wanted us all to dedicate our lives and careers solely to the solution of the riddle created by her ever-changing symptoms, to find and name whatever it was that lurked deep inside her and made her so miserable. The core problem, however, boiled down to this—there just wasn't a whole lot physically wrong with Rosemary. At least not a whole lot that wasn't easily explainable by taking the mileage on her personal odometer plus the reading on her bathroom scale, then simply doing the math.

One thing Rosemary absolutely never experienced was anything common. Not even the common cold, which is where my involvement in her life began.

My first encounter with Rosemary should have clued me in to what lay in store for our relationship. I opened the exam room door that first day, and there she sat perched on the exam table, fidgeting like a chubby robin in a birdbath. Before I was able to greet her and introduce myself properly, she started into the never-ending list of everything that was wrong with her. No matter what I asked about—on the rare occasions that I actually completed a sentence—it was not working right, and I soon learned that, with her, taking a long history was not a great idea. At best it would only extend our visit by twenty minutes and confuse things all the more.

Rosemary was dressed in what I would find out later was her "coming to see the doctor" uniform: a shiny brown-and-orange acetate housedress with what looked like a large campaign button affixed to the left collar. Closer inspection revealed it to be a button with a picture of Saint Christopher on it. I knew he was the patron saint of travelers, but I wasn't aware he had been assigned jurisdiction over geriatrics. I never figured out the point of that ever-present button. Was it intended to intimidate the doctor, remind us all of who was really in the driver's seat? Or did it just serve as a good luck charm, a poultice to fend off evil physicians? For reasons only Rosemary could say, it was there for every visit, as was her husband, John. He was a semimute Jack Sprat of a man who always stood in the corner of the room, I think so no one could sneak up on him. During our visits he kept his eyes focused on the floor, working his hands nervously around the brim of his '40s-style hat. It was almost as if he had a force field around him that repelled all intruders. If you got too close to him, he would step back and reposition himself in order to reestablish the five feet of personal space he apparently required.

Rosemary's complaints kept rolling. Her back was killing her, she couldn't "hold her water," and she was sure she had had TB, malaria, and salmonella in the past. I was tempted to ask her the trick question about whether her stools sometimes glowed in the dark, but resisted. The only thing in Rosemary's estimation that worked well was her heart. "My mother always told me I had a strong heart," was a comment I could count on hearing at nearly every visit. In that first conversation I learned some other things about Rosemary's health. She was convinced that the world was conspiring to get her. She suspected that she was being slowly poisoned by the air she breathed (pollution), the food she ate (preservatives), her furnace (carbon monoxide), as well as the radon in the basement and the high-tension wires behind her house. Oops, forgot to mention all her neighbor's cell phones. ("Don't you know those waves go right through your brain!") It was as if she had taken every TV newsmagazine "inside report" on health dangers and personally applied it to her own life. Except of course the ones about diet and exercise. She fretted about the use of her microwave oven because she read somewhere that the microwaves neutralized all the vitamins in her food. As a result, she stocked a host of home remedies and vitamin preparations that would have required a small U-Haul to carry around had she ever traveled, which she did not because of—yes, you guessed it—how dangerous the roads were. None of this, however, is what brought Rosemary in to see me that first day. She was there that day for a cold.

"I'm choking, I can hardly breathe, I'm telling you," Rosemary squawked in an odd voice, vaguely reminiscent of the sound you make after taking a hit on a helium balloon. Her husband kept his post in the corner, never looking up or establishing eye contact. He just stood there, feverishly fingering the worn brim of that fedora and muttering an ongoing counterconversation to each of Rosemary's complaints. For example, Rosemary would talk about her choking, and he would mutter under his breath, "Tell him about your headaches, Rosemary. Be sure and tell him about your headaches." Rosemary, paying him no attention, would talk about her cough, and he would mumble, "Tell him about your legs, Rosemary. Don't forget to tell him about those legs."

I eventually came to doubt that concern for her headaches or her legs or any of the rest of her symptoms was John's primary motivation for being there. I think he was just looking for some kind of bunker into which he could retreat when her barrage of complaints must have continued at home. At least he'd be able to say that she had already mentioned it to the doctor, so don't worry. Utterly ignoring his interjections, their verbal tennis match continued as she embellished the sad story of her cold.

"The phlegm is choking me, Doctor. I can't take it anymore. You have to help me." While she talked full steam, I proceeded with an examination—holding the tongue depressor in her mouth just a little longer than truly necessary just to get a moment's break from her monologue. I found little evidence of anything other than an obese older woman with a head cold.

Glad to have arrived at such a benign conclusion, I gave her the happy news, but by the expression on her face it was plain that she interpreted it as anything but. "Rosemary, I'm going to run a few tests to check out some of the other complaints you have." I suspected that Rosemary was well on her way to breaking the Medicare bank single-handedly, but sometimes a "normal" on a lab report can purchase a little peace of mind. "In the meantime I'm going to give you a prescription to help with that congestion. We'll call you about the results as soon as they come back."

I turned to leave the room, a little relieved to be moving on to the next patient. But no sooner had my hand touched the doorknob than I heard a bloodcurdling scream behind me and turned to find Rosemary midway through what appeared to be a stop-drop-and-roll. She had apparently taken one giant leap for mankind off the exam table and missed the step on the end. In an instant there she was, rolled up into a ball in the corner of the room at her husband's feet—who, by the way, just stood there wide-eyed, immobilized by the fact that she had penetrated his force field. The only thing moving were his fingers, around the brim of that hat, at twice their normal speed. I rushed over to her and, unassisted, hoisted her back onto the table. Then we x-rayed her from stem to stern. Her x-rays were normal; her extra padding had apparently saved her from significant injury to anything other than her pride.

I received one or two calls a day from Rosemary for the next ten days telling me just exactly how she was "choking to death" that particular day and how it was different from how she had been "choking to death" the day before and how she needed some new medicine right away. After three office visits and multiple phone calls (during one of which I actually heard myself say, "Rosemary, if you can say the words 'I'm choking to death'. . . you're not!"), Rosemary did eventually survive that cold. Not, of course, without multiple complaints about how long it took us to get her feeling better and her deep suspicion that we were missing something. Despite the unreasonableness of her expectations, I couldn't lose the feeling of responsibility. I think all physicians have a bit of a savior complex skulking about inside somewhere, and I must admit I am no exception. Despite her tirades about how wrong every other doctor had been, I remained confident that somehow, with enough care and wisdom and kindness and time, I would be able to get to the bottom of what was really generating Rosemary's problems. I would be the one who would break the spell and put her back on the road to health.

I don't know if you could say we became friends over the next year and a half, but we were at least traveling companions. Like two people forced by fate to share the same seat on a long bus ride, we grew used to one another. Maybe with some people that's as good as it gets. And though she never gave me any sense that she appreciated anything I did for her, or for that matter had any real faith in what I told her, Rosemary became a regular feature on my schedule. At the time I thought about 90 percent of how I felt about her was irritation, but I think there was more. Inside me there remained this need to help her somehow, to free her just a little bit from the chains she carried. The fear of being ill was crippling her more than any real illness would have. It was an ever-growing fixation that left less and less room for real living. But her chains were very powerful, and as the months went by, each visit with her became just a little bit more absurd than the last.

A year or so after that first visit came the fateful day when I looked down at my schedule and saw this looking back at me: "Rosemary T.—Check female problem."

My nurse and I looked at each other, and both of us shook our heads. Before long I saw my nurse coming down the hall with Rosemary close behind her, her husband apparently opting out of this one . . . not a good sign. I gathered my courage and my nurse Laurie, and with a mutual deep breath we opened the exam-room door unprepared for what greeted us. There was Rosemary, on her own initiative, lying on her back on the exam table, her black orthopedic wedgies jammed tightly into the stirrups.

She started complaining the moment the door opened. "I don't know what it is, Doctor, but something feels really, really terrible down there. It's irritating me and I'm all itchy. It's awful, just awful." Rather than go through the hassle of getting her down from the "ready position," only to have to get her back up there, I decided to go straight to the exam. I put on my gloves, sat on the exam stool, pushed back her dress, and as soon as I did, found myself face to face with the problem. There, affixed to her left buttock, was a price tag—all alone—reminiscent of a postage stamp smacked on the surface of the moon.

$1.97

As big as life. I stared at the price tag a moment then reflexively took the Q-Tip swab that was in my right hand and simply pointed to the tag to highlight it for my nurse who was poised over my right shoulder. Laurie saw the price tag and went into a convulsion of badly camouflaged cough-laughter, then stumbled behind me, made some sort of lame excuse about needing a sip of water, and fled the exam room.

So there we were, just Rosemary, me, Saint Christopher, and the price tag. I was lost for a moment in a sea of questions: How could it possibly have gotten there? Why didn't she feel it and remove it herself? And how was I going to tell her what it was without making her feel silly? I ended up with no good answer to any of the three questions, so I simply removed the price tag, stuck it in her chart, and told Rosemary that I had solved the problem. Rosemary reached down and found that, indeed, the irritant was gone. If her momentary thankfulness had been the measure, you would have thought I had just cured cancer. I wondered later if she thought, *Finally a problem with a solution.* With some significant effort, I un-wedged her shoes from the stirrups and she got down off the table. Then, while struggling to step back into her undies with her shoes still on, without missing a beat, she proceeded right into her next complaint—her back.

Our relationship came to an abrupt end several weeks later when finally, after months of complaints with little substance, I suggested to Rosemary in the most gentle tones I could manage that maybe, just maybe, there was an emotional component tying together all these physical complaints. If not causing some of them, certainly it was making them worse. Little did I know that *psychiatrist* was the magic word that had consistently ended Rosemary's relationship with each of her previous physicians. Suggesting that her symptoms weren't purely physical said to her that I no longer believed what she said about her ailments, and that would not be tolerated. It hadn't really occurred to me until that moment, but in some ways her symptoms were really all she had. She shouted at me, "Oh, a psychiatrist. That's what you're suggesting, isn't it? Well, I'm not crazy! What good can a psychiatrist do when you're practically dying? My mother took me to a psychiatrist when I was a girl, and it didn't help one single bit." There were tears in her eyes as she spit out this last sentence and pushed past me into the hallway. I was flabbergasted, really. I couldn't imagine the significance she attached to what I had just said. The visit concluded with me handing the card of one of my counseling colleagues to her husband as he pursued her down the hall. He just looked at it and stuffed it into his coat pocket. I think he had played this scene several times before.

I was sadder than I expected to be, watching Rosemary huff out of the office that day, and I was surprised by how much I missed her. Rosemary on my schedule had been a weekly occurrence, and somehow a week without her usual cavalcade of complaints seemed incomplete. She had become a constant in my life—dependable, consistent, reliable—like a crotchety old friend, whom you think you'll be glad to be rid of. Yet once they're gone, you discover how much a part of your world they had become and how much comfort you had derived from their just being there.

I was also saddened by the fact that I wasn't able to deliver the message she so desperately needed to hear: that her worth as a person, her deserving compassion and attention, didn't need to hang on her being stricken with some mysterious illness. I wanted somehow to convey to her that she mattered to God and the rest of us with or without a terrible disease. That message just never got through, and I came to believe it most likely never would. Rosemary's pattern was so deeply ingrained. Her comment about her mother had landed like a punch. There was a reason Rosemary was who she was. I was sure there was a painful story there, but I doubted anyone would ever know it. I think her myriad of mostly imagined illnesses gave both her and her husband a raison d'être—a reason to live, a battle to fight. Her symptoms were their shared enemy, their common bond, and it turned their life together into a kind of journey, a quest for an answer always just beyond their grasp. As I thought about them on that journey, mostly alone, mostly afraid, it occurred to me why she wore her Saint Christopher's button.

POSTSCRIPT

Rosemary bounced through several other doctors in town over the next eight years. Whenever I saw her name on the hospital census, I would ask the nurses how she was doing and got the same rolled eyes and "Oh, you too?" kind of response from just about everyone. She was never with any one doctor for much more than a year. Although there was one part of me that pretended to be glad just to be rid of her craziness, I couldn't get rid of a vague sense of failure whenever I thought of her. It occurred to me that Rosemary had gotten something tragically turned around, something maybe we all lose sight of sometimes. The storms that batter us arise mostly from within, while the shelter we seek is most often found without. Rosemary could never see that. She remained convinced to the end that there was something external that caused her heart to be so troubled. Ironically, Rosemary died suddenly of a heart attack—the one thing she had never complained about, the one thing she was sure was okay.

As for Sadie, she took a slow, steady, downhill course into senile dementia. With each visit I found just a little less of her there to greet me. At each visit her husband's doting care seemed more loving, less condescending, and more appropriate. Maybe all along he knew better than I did what was coming. My primary relationship slowly shifted to Frank, both of us watching helplessly as Sadie gradually faded away. It was an excruciating exit, and between our discussions about her medications and care, I would catch fleeting glimpses of what tough old Frank was feeling. It was mostly pain. The pain of the one who must remain behind. The pain of losing his winter companion, being left to face that season alone. In the end, the pain of never being able to tell his wife good-bye. It took no small amount of effort to finally get Frank to agree to place his wife in a nursing facility when her daily needs became too much for him to handle. He spent hours with her every day, without fail, until her death almost five years later. As far as I know, she never stopped smiling.

TAMMY

There was a mix of fear and "foreign soil" about them that made the word *immigrants* flash through my mind when I first saw them huddled together at the examination table. The dark-haired young man stood very close to the slight young girl, protecting her as she sat cloistered against his shoulder. She was shy and uneasy. Her over-long blond bangs seemed intentionally designed to help her avoid eye contact. He looked as if he had stepped out of another decade, with his black leather jacket and long dark hair, trying to hide his anxiety behind his machismo. When teamed with his youth, it came across more as comic than intimidating. He did all the talking at first.

"We're here to see if you can deliver our baby," he blurted out awkwardly. It really sounded more like a challenge than a request.

For the next several minutes I tried to put them at ease, get a little information, talk about the process, the prenatal visit schedule, etc., and just let their story evolve. Their names were Tammy and David. They were not married; she was pregnant and seventeen years old. The news of the pregnancy had caused something just shy of a nuclear meltdown at her house. Her parents had never approved of the relationship. Her father exploded with the news of the pregnancy, and "either he goes, or you go" had been the result. Tammy chose David. As I looked at them together, there was something endearing, a sort of "us against the world" quality that engaged me right away. That first day they seemed like two children caught alone in a storm. I guess in many ways that is exactly what they were. What they didn't know was that the storm had just barely begun.

When Tammy did finally speak, her voice seemed garbled, all thick and nasal and swallowed sounding. As I started the physical exam, I asked Tammy if there had been any change in her voice recently. She said yes, that this had been going on for several months. She thought she just had a bad cold or a sinus infection that wouldn't go away. I asked her to open her mouth and experienced that thing that happens to a doctor when he finds something undeniable. Whether it's a lump or a sound or a shadow on an x-ray, suddenly you're looking at an omen of what is to come, the slow-motion descent of the first leaf down in autumn. It feels like someone has just blown a flashbulb in your face—it's a moment or two before you can see clearly again. Immediately I could see their story turning down a whole new path, a difficult dark path. I knew that Tammy had something pushing down out of her sinus area, distorting her soft palate, the part that moves when we speak. I was pretty sure I was looking at a tumor.

I had to think of how to put this. I began to lecture myself inside. *Now be careful. Don't be too drastic. If you do they'll think you're an alarmist. You'll scare them off and they'll end up dismissing this and she'll be in even greater danger than she's in already.*

There is nothing worse than having to deliver bad news on a first visit. Especially when it is directly contrary to what the patient is expecting. But they needed to understand that there was a big problem here, and we all needed to know the exact nature of it for Tammy's sake and the baby's.

I finished the rest of her exam, which showed no additional problems other than a weight gain that was a little less than expected.

"Tammy, as far as the baby is concerned, everything seems just fine. The baby is growing at just the rate we would think he should, the heart tones are good, and the date at which you first felt movement seems right on." I hated to erase her smile with what I needed to say next. "It's you I'm concerned about though. There is something—I don't know what—pushing down against your palate. It's the reason your voice has changed. It's some kind of fullness, the exact nature of which I can't tell you right now. It could be a lot of different things, Tammy. An infection possibly, a growth of some type, maybe." I could sense her retreating. "The sooner we know exactly what it is the sooner we can get you appropriate treatment and make it go away. I have a colleague; he's located just up the street from here. He's an ear, nose, and throat specialist, and I'd like to send you right up there to get his opinion."

"Growth? What do you mean? You mean like a tumor or something? Everything's gonna be all right isn't it, like it's nothing serious or anything is it?" David immediately jumped in, feeling a threat. It was his way of protecting her, as if his words could somehow bend reality back into place.

"I don't know the answer to that yet, David. That's what we need to find out."

I knew that unless David bought into this we were going to end up with serious delays. He needed to be part of the process right now. Standing by as a spectator would make him feel insecure and powerless and he'd be more likely to do something counterproductive.

"David, can you get Tammy up to the other doctor's office today? I will also need you to call me back this afternoon and tell me how everything went and what he said."

Now, obviously my ENT associate would call me as soon as he had any information, but David needed a role in all this, and I was hoping that this one, a sort of scout, would be enough to make him feel like he was in some kind of control.

·"Sure, sure. What's the number?"

I wrote my home number on the back of my card, gave it to David, then stepped out of the room and called the specialist. He was able to work them in that afternoon.

I got a call back right away. The specialist was very concerned by what he saw on his exam. Tammy definitely had some type of mass bearing down out of the sinus area. It was strange; he had never seen anything quite like it. He took some initial biopsies in his office and would call back as soon as he received a report.

The report took longer than expected because I think the pathologist had difficulty believing what he was seeing. It was a tumor and it was malignant, but it was a very rare type for this kind of a patient—something called a Burkitt's lymphoma, apparently involving the sinus area only. I spent a lot of time on the phone with David about what was happening each step of the way as the information was confirmed. Yes, it was malignant, but treatable. No, it wasn't anywhere else. No, she couldn't give it to the baby. We all agreed that with the combination of the pregnancy and the rarity of the tumor, Tammy would be best cared for at a specialty referral hospital in the city.

Over the next several months most of my information about Tammy came through copies of letters from the doctors at the referral hospital. They agreed with the diagnosis, found no evidence of tumor anywhere except the sinus area, and proceeded with a five-drug chemotherapy regimen. Tammy was one-third of the way through her pregnancy when the treatments began. I could tell by the tone of the letters that she had been sternly counseled to abort the baby, but she steadfastly refused.

I was surprised for some reason. Although I didn't really know her, it just seemed uncharacteristic of the shy little girl I had met that day in the office. She seemed so very meek and retiring, but there was apparently something more inside than I was able to see at first.

The letters from the medical center were full of what is nicely known in the medical world as "cover your butt" statements, like "likelihood of deformity," "adverse effect on the fetus," almost "certain developmental impact on the child." But despite what must have amounted to pleading on the part of the high-powered team of specialists caring for her, Tammy saw this situation as clearly and simply as I think it could be seen. To her there were possible problems on one hand and certain death on the other. She had chosen life for herself and could do no less for her child, whatever that meant.

I thought about Tammy often during the next several weeks. My only link to her was the reports I received and a rare phone call from her boyfriend. Tammy found a strength that surprised almost everyone. She was going to beat this thing; she was going to give her child a chance at life; he was going to be okay. She was going to have faith in this frightening place, even if that faith at times felt like little more than a humming in the darkness of her room.

There was a strange symbiosis going on here. In one way she was saving her baby; in another way it was her baby saving her. The complicating pregnancy provided Tammy with the motivation she needed to keep at it, to endure the fear and the side effects of the chemotherapy and the dehumanizing impact of the medical center. Each of those things, I think, had its own peculiar toxicity. I found out later that Tammy's mother and her much younger sister and brother visited several times during her stay in the hospital, and although her father remained somewhat distant, there was some healing going on there as well.

Tammy completed twelve weeks of chemotherapy, and when it was over, all evidence of the tumor had disappeared. It had simply melted away. The department of oncology completed a final series of x-rays and other tests, then set up follow-up visits for Tammy every four weeks for the next several months. The tumor was so rare, everyone felt more insecure than usual about predicting the long-term future. But for now, everyone was just thankful she was free of any evidence of tumor. The letters from the doctors in the OB-GYN department caring for her pregnancy continued to be peppered with phrases of concern about the health of her baby, although all objective testing seemed to indicate no observable problems.

The next time I saw Tammy was six weeks before her due date. It surprised me to see her there, again with David. We exchanged greetings, and I told her how glad I was about the good news from the other doctors. This time it was Tammy who spoke.

"Dr. Judge, please, will you deliver my baby?" I must have looked puzzled because she continued right away. "I don't trust those doctors downtown. They wanted to kill it. I can't go back there. I'm having nightmares about it. I can't . . . I don't trust them."

Inside I could feel my defenses activating. My practical side started to get a little nervous. Tammy's was in no sense a "clean" case—family discord, an unmarried mother, a hostile boyfriend, a malignant tumor, major chemotherapy. Why was I even considering this? It was just the kind of case lawyers advise doctors to avoid like the plague. I could visualize my malpractice lawyer looking at me someday and saying, "What on earth were you thinking?" Was I just being stupid? I could have easily stepped away and 99 percent of the world would have applauded my wisdom. The problem was that I was looking straight into the face of the other 1 percent. And when I looked at her, and I thought of her own bravery and what she had been through and what still lay ahead, there was simply no other option.

Before I knew it I heard myself say, "Listen, Tammy, I need to talk to your OB doctors to make sure they don't foresee any special-care needs for the delivery. If they feel that the delivery itself is likely to be basically uncomplicated, then I will be glad to do the delivery." She smiled and reached forward and grasped my hand, and for a moment I remembered why I had become a doctor.

There was an almost audible sigh of relief on the other end of the phone when I posed the question to the doctors caring for Tammy's pregnancy at the referral hospital. They did not see that the delivery itself would be complicated; they only suggested that I have a neonatologist on call in case there was any problem with the baby. I could practically hear them snickering "Sucker" in the background as I put down the receiver.

It was David, Tammy, and me in the delivery room three weeks later. Tammy had gone into labor ten days early. Her delivery was amazingly fast and uncomplicated. She delivered a beautiful baby boy, blond, and as Tammy said when she first saw him . . . "perfect." We had the neonatologist look him over, just as a precaution, and he agreed that the baby looked completely healthy.

The second day after delivery I sat on the end of Tammy's bed, and we talked together for a good while about the delivery and her baby and the miracle of it all working out. We talked about how sometimes God is most easily seen at work in our lives when everything seems to be going wrong. She nodded and smiled, and I remember thinking how different this young woman was from the person who came into my office that first day. There was a strength, an energy, almost a glow. Moms the first couple of days after delivery are not always at their best, yet Tammy looked absolutely radiant. I remember thinking I was looking at someone who had run the race and knew she had run it well.

"Looks like you made the right decision, Tammy. You've got a beautiful healthy baby. Congratulations," I said.

"He is beautiful, isn't he? What if I had listened to those doctors down at the other hospital? He was worth it you know, worth all of it," she said, never taking her eyes off her son.

I sat there a moment watching them. She looked almost like a Byzantine Madonna, her gaunt face and long blond hair, holding her sleeping newborn son. I freeze-framed the picture in my memory.

I got up. "Tomorrow we'll get practical and talk about all the going-home instructions. The fun has just begun you know. There's lots of work ahead."

She simply smiled, looked up, and said thank you. Maybe the most sincere and simple thank you I had ever received. It was a gift.

It was Saturday, so I was home that afternoon, swimming with the kids when I received a frantic call from the postpartum nurse. All I got was Tammy's name, respiratory arrest, cardiac care unit, come right away. I got into some jeans, jumped into the car, and sped to the hospital. When I arrived at the coronary care unit, I recognized all the telltale signs of a recent code blue: yards and yards of EKG tape strewn everywhere, the defibrillator paddles sitting all askew, respiratory therapists and nurses all huddled around whispering. The cardiologist filled me in on the details. Tammy, out of nowhere, had gotten suddenly short of breath and complained of chest pain. The nurses called the on-call physician who had ordered a chest x-ray and blood gases, worrying appropriately that she could have had a blood clot to the lung, a described complication after delivery with some women. But no sooner had these been done then the shortness of breath became acutely worse. They called the cardiologist who was at the hospital. He arrived at her room at the same time as the x-ray results, which demonstrated that the sac around Tammy's heart was filling with fluid, massively, and the pressure from the fluid was pressing on her heart, preventing it from beating. He had done an immediate procedure to remove the fluid from the sac right there, and then moved her to the cardiac care unit. Just as she arrived at the unit, her heart's electrical rhythm began to act bizarrely, and she went into a ventricular tachycardia. Despite every effort at resuscitation, she had died just moments before I arrived.

I walked slowly over to her intensive care room, glassed all the way around, open on one side to the center unit. As I looked at her, for a moment she was Sleeping Beauty. I walked into the room in disbelief. She lay on the bed, ET tube still in, IVs still hung. A palpable silence all around. I touched her cold hand, choking back the emotion that threatened to take over, and just stood there for a few moments, dazed. A rising tide of *why*s engulfed me. *Why* after everything she has been through, after beating all the odds, *why* now? *Why* her? She barely had a chance at living.

The nurse must have been talking to me, but I missed it at first.

"Dr. Judge, I said the family is here; they are in the consultation room. They don't know she died. Do you want to talk to them?"

"What? Yes, sure, sure. Tell them I'll be right there."

I steadied myself a moment, then got ready for what had

to happen next. I started to detach, uncouple my own emotions from the situation. It was the only way I could make it through. I walked into the small room, and I am sure that everything about me screamed the answer to their question. Tammy's mother, a pretty lady in her late thirties who looked a lot like Tammy, sat with Tammy's sister and brother. Her father stood against the back wall.

"Tammy had a cardiac arrest about an hour ago. Every attempt was made to resuscitate her, but all our efforts failed. Tammy didn't make it." It was as if the room suddenly burst into flames. There was bedlam. Her father collapsed into the chair beside him and covered a face full of horror and disbelief, as any chance of saying the things he wanted to say to her evaporated. Tammy's younger brother and sister screamed and rushed to their mother, who held them tightly, rocking back and forth, weeping. No one knew where David was.

"How, how could it happen? We just talked with her this morning; she was fine."

I knew what to expect. The denial, the anger, the bargaining. But I was caught off guard. I guess I just didn't expect to be going through it with them. I could spit back the stages of grief on request, but no one tells you that they all come in five minutes and keep coming for years afterward, and that you as the doctor get dragged through them all with the family. I wanted to sob with them, to do my own grieving, but I told myself it was stupid. I was just the doctor, not the family, and it wouldn't help anyone.

I walked through all the events of the morning, one by one. There is a hard kind of comfort that comes for a family in knowing every detail, no matter how minuscule and meaningless. There is a kind of comfort for the doctor in stating them. It creates a space, I suppose. And so I went through everything I could tell them, then heard myself say, "We don't know exactly why this happened. She had a chest x-ray a month ago that was completely normal." There had been no evidence of any heart problems throughout her previous hospitalization.

"I can only imagine how desperately hard this must be for you, but I need to ask your permission to have an autopsy done. Hopefully, we'll get some kind of answer from this." Words fail to describe how it felt to ask this at that moment. As if all the rest was not painful enough. I felt dirty for some reason, as if I was more interested in getting some t's crossed, some i's dotted than in the human agony unfolding around me. For that moment I hated what I did for a living. I couldn't imagine I had been stupid enough to choose a profession that required you to ask such a thing of parents who had just lost a child. Tammy's father gave his permission for the autopsy.

I looked at the family and told them how sorry I was about their daughter's death. About how much she loved her baby, how very brave she was. After a few moments to allow them to gain composure, I led the family into the unit to see Tammy and say their own good-byes. I stood in the corner as her parents bent over and embraced their daughter one last time. It was like watching the scene from thirty feet up, like I was suspended above the room, not actually in it. They cried and touched her, and after a while I left them alone.

I went to the nurses' station and asked the nurses to be sure to have her father sign the permission papers for the autopsy. And I walked through the hospital corridor and out to my car. The whole trip home all I remember was anger, probably because it was the only feeling I was very good at. Anger at everything and everyone. At myself, for being stupid enough to get involved with this from the beginning. There was nothing in the world that was worth going through what had just happened, nothing. I wanted to scream. Anger at the injustice, the futility of it all, the just plain stupid waste. The whole story felt like it was without redemption. Where was God? Because if he wasn't in this, somewhere, then maybe he just wasn't anywhere.

I drove home too fast and swung the car into the driveway. I opened the car door and was suddenly in a new world. The color began to seep back in. I could hear my three daughters' laughter in the pool in the backyard, and for a moment I stood there shaking, choking back what threatened to bring me to my knees. I held on to the handle of that car door, clutching it desperately, knowing that if I let go too soon, I might be swept away. Then I walked into the house, put my swimsuit on, walked back to the pool, and dove in. It was surreal, to be swimming with my family on a bright sunny day, moments after leaving Tammy and her family. Three miles was all that separated one universe from the other.

I told myself a familiar lie. I told myself that my feelings, the emotions inside, could be put off, dealt with later. That it was, in fact, smart to do this. That they could be stuffed down and pulled back out at some time less risky, more convenient. Some time when it felt safer. It's been said that "dreams deferred dry up like raisins in the sun." Well, I can tell you from experience, feelings deferred share a similar fate.

I think I already knew that, even then. I think I already knew that my buried emotions could not be resurrected in their previous form. If I ever did get around to unearthing them, they would be dried up and shriveled and unrecognizable. What I was really doing was protecting myself—it was all about self-defense. Deferring the feelings was just a form of denial. I didn't know what to do with them, and not knowing for a doctor, for this doctor, was just not an option. So I pretended I would feel them later.

There was another lie that I told myself—that I could limit this habit of putting off feelings to just my professional life. But if I had been brave enough for introspection, I would have seen even then that putting off my feelings was becoming an overall pattern. It was a kind of numbing that was beginning to invade my entire life. The numbness, for some reason, felt good and strangely safe. I can only imagine that it must be, in some ways, similar to what drives an alcoholic when he drinks. It's a kind of anesthetic, really. I was functioning, always well-functioning, but there was day by day less and less of anyone real inside. A hollow Tin Man who had lost sight of the Emerald City.

The next morning I arrived at the hospital pathology lab just as the autopsy results were being dictated. The pathologist looked at me and just shook his head.

"You're not going to believe this, Jim, but I found no evidence of any tumor anywhere in her whole body . . . until we got to her heart. Her heart was 80 percent infiltrated with tumor. I've never seen anything like it. Jim, it's nothing short of a miracle she didn't arrest sooner than she did. I can't imagine how she got through labor."

Slowly a series of events began to take on a logic. More than logic. A loving direction. Tammy enduring the chemotherapy, going into labor almost two weeks early, the unusually easy character of the labor itself, the miracle of a perfect child. I saw a series of miracles lining up and pointing straight somewhere. I wondered whether her arrival in my office months before and what I was wrestling with right then were two more points on the same line. But I was still angry and refused to look in the direction it all pointed. Tammy was dead, and the acute pain of that and the sheer waste of it obscured everything else.

Three days later I was talking with her family at the funeral home. I hated being there. I always felt strangely out of place. Maybe what I hated most about it was the awkwardness of being introduced as the "doctor of the deceased," and the feeling of failure that came with it. I spoke to her parents again about Tammy's great strength, about the conviction she had that her purpose was to give birth to her son. Unimaginable for someone who was little more than a child herself.

As I walked toward the door of the funeral home to leave, there, standing at the door, was a familiar face. It was Nellie, an older lady who attended the same church I did. She had been widowed a long time back, and she and her husband were legends around town. I had never known her husband, who had been the chaplain of a local college, but everyone who had known him had a story about him. My favorite was about his regular long morning walks around town. He was known to stop in front of the houses of people he knew and just stand there and pray out loud for them. As I looked at

Nellie, I flashed to that story about her husband and wished deep inside that he was still around and would come and stand in front of my house. Nellie was herself a bit of a crazy saint. One part Mother Teresa, one part Mammy Yokum. I couldn't imagine what connection she had here.

She had seen me come in and felt an urge to tell me something. Every conversation I had ever had with Nellie had this same sense of her revealing something secret and amazing. Her eyes dancing with a kind of holy fire, in hushed and hurried tones, she told me that the night after Tammy had given birth, she and a friend came to do hospital visitation. Someone from the church had given them Tammy's name. From the first moment of their visit, Nellie said, it was as if Tammy had been waiting for them. She had all kinds of spiritual questions, questions that were sincere and honest. Somehow, unimaginably, this ancient saint connected with this unwed seventeen-year-old mother. Maybe that's one of the miracles that all saints can do. Maybe when saints speak, it's a different, more familiar voice people hear. Anyway, by the time their conversation ended, Tammy told them she wanted to know God. She wanted to start a new life with him beside her. They prayed together that night, the ancient saint and the young mother. Nellie returned the next night, only to be told Tammy had died.

I stood there trembling, assaulted by this ruthless grace. It was the mortar that held the whole story together, held each of us together. Tammy was at peace, complete and perfect. Nellie had been the agent of one more miracle. And then there was the extravagant, nearly prodigal grace poured out on me. What if Nellie had not come to the funeral home at the exact time I did? I don't think until I showed up she even knew I was Tammy's doctor. What if I had never heard this final chapter? Would that have made God less loving, less just, less merciful? How many other times in my life would I not be handed the final piece to a puzzle, and simply be asked to believe that it existed? Asked to believe and wait.

I just stared at Nellie, holding this last piece to the beautiful puzzle that was Tammy, the one I were sure was lost forever, if it had even existed. I felt as if I were standing over the table, holding it in my hand, torn between putting it in its place and letting the incompleteness and the tension linger just a moment longer. I knew that once I pressed it down into place something lovely would appear. But at the same time, something else would come to an end; the not knowing and the wonder and the mystery would be gone. The opportunity for faith. There's something beautiful about the incomplete, something almost holy.

POSTSCRIPT

David's grief was unrestrained. He made threats to the nurses about coming back and taking the child before we "killed it too." The hospital staff put a fictitious name on the baby's crib and watched very carefully for those several days that followed. Security reported someone they thought was David on the hospital grounds, but he didn't enter the building. I never saw David again. There was no way he could raise a child by himself, and I think he knew it.

Tammy's son, Danny, was adopted by his grandparents, who were only in their late thirties at the time of their daughter's death. I was Danny's doctor until he was eight years old. When he was ten, packages from his father began to arrive, and over the next several years their connection deepened. David, by this time, was married, had a good job, and was living in another state. He very much wanted to know his son. Eventually, Danny's custody was transferred to his father, and Danny now lives with his dad.

When I contacted Tammy's mother to give her a copy of the manuscript she gave me an important piece to this story I did not have. The first day of Tammy's chemotherapy the doctors warned her the treatment would almost certainly induce a spontaneous abortion. Her mother stayed with Tammy late into that first terrible night, but at about 1:30 AM she went home to her other children. When she returned the next morning, she found Tammy sitting up in bed smiling. Her mother asked what had happened, and Tammy replied, "I'm not afraid anymore, Mom. Last night Jesus told me that my baby is going to be all right."

That baby is now a teenager. He is gifted in many ways: a talented drummer, an accomplished wrestler, an honor-roll student. I promised myself in those days after Tammy's death that I would write this story and give it to Danny one day. I sent him the story shortly before the book's publication, hoping it might in some small way let him know something of his mother's great love and courage, and of the providence that watched over him before he was born. A providence that watches over him still.

A year after Tammy's death, I stopped delivering babies.

MANDY

I had the privilege of playing a small supportive role in a miracle once—a miracle named Mandy, who in her whole life never really smiled or sang a song, never spoke a word. Never as far as I know even moved an arm or a leg as a matter of her own will. But as unlikely as it might seem, she taught me more about what it is to be loved and what it is to be real than just about any other patient I can think of.

Mandy's brain, for all intents and purposes, had been terribly miswired. Nothing seemed to be connected to what it was supposed to be connected to. We had no evidence that she could either see or hear. Her movements seemed random; even the most primitive reflexes were lacking. We think she was aware of being held, but even that could have been wishful thinking. Her profound internal derangement stood in stark contrast to her outward appearance. Her chubby cheeks were a constant sort of English schoolgirl pink, which when combined with her blond corn silk hair, gave her the appearance of a Rubenesque cherub about to take flight at any moment.

It happened to me the first time I examined Mandy, and again at almost every visit. As I bent over her that first morning, listening to her heart through my stethoscope, I found myself being drawn to her eyes. She didn't have that searching, frantic, back-and-forth motion many blind people have. Her gaze was fixed, as if she was seeing something, someplace, someone the rest of us could not, something she could not take her eyes off of. There was a drawing darkness to her eyes that seemed to pull me in. Not a frightening darkness, but rather a warm, mysteriously familiar darkness, like the welcomed blanketing darkness of your own bedroom as you slip across the border that separates waking from dreams. Her eyes seemed to contain a universe all their own, and when you looked down into them, you half expected to see tiny galaxies spinning within. There was an overwhelming sense of peace about her. Looking down at her made me feel that she possessed some great essential secret, a secret set to music. I strained to make out its melody, unable to shake the feeling that if I could just be quiet enough I might remember where I had heard it before.

A strange kind of calm engulfed me at that first visit, a weariness released. I felt a quietness take over, a sense of peace pervade; that day's troubles just seemed to melt away. I had the feeling that I had come into the presence of someone almost holy. All the emotions I thought I would feel, like compassion or its poor relation pity, went missing. Instead I felt myself calmed and wanting only to hold her. As far as I could tell, it wasn't a result of how she looked or anything she did. It wasn't external at all. It was something that happened *in* me. I have talked to others who came close to Mandy, and they describe a very similar experience. All of this within the power of a sightless little child who without never indicated she knew I was in the room, but within somehow assured me that I was the only person on earth.

My part in Mandy's story began several months before her birth, in a nonprofessional setting. My wife and I were speaking to a mother-of-preschoolers group that was led by Mandy's soon-to-be mother, Susan. I was Susan's personal physician, and she and her husband, Marshall, were high up on the list of people I wished I knew better. There was a sense of direction about them that was attractive. A steadiness. They seemed to be able to draw all the good things out of the evangelical subculture they were a part of and somehow kept it from smothering or stifling the life inside. Bottom line—they managed to stay real, and because that was a front upon which I was doing personal battle right then, it probably made me like them all the more.

Susan caught us in the hallway outside when we were finished speaking that morning and surprised us with a good news–bad news scenario we weren't prepared for. She was pregnant, and the amniocentesis had shown that the baby would be a girl, their third.

Susan, knowing we had three girls, asked how we had dealt with that disappointment. My wife and I both fumbled for an answer, I think in part because of how the question was phrased. "The disappointment of having three girls," instead of the disappointment of not having a son. The three of us talked about it for a while, but my wife and I both had a hard time relating to the level of emotion she was experiencing, and the whole encounter left me with a vague feeling there was more to the question than we ever got to that morning.

Susan's pregnancy was uncomplicated, and several months later she delivered her baby at a local hospital. Her newborn daughter's problems, previously unsuspected, were immediately apparent. Her daughter was microcephalic, meaning the baby's head was disproportionately small. Alone, this could mean anything from nothing to profound retardation. Susan left the hospital knowing only that her baby was not normal. At two weeks of age Mandy had her first seizure. Because the delivery was not at a hospital where I saw newborns, my first contact with Mandy did not occur until she was more than a month old and had already amassed a dramatic medical file. She had been seen by multiple specialists already, and with each new consultation came a progressively more dismal forecast. For reasons that remain a mystery even now, Mandy was profoundly brain damaged. She had cataracts and although there was hope that with their removal she might be able to see, we found out only after the operation that there was no connection between her eyes and the part of the brain responsible for sight. There was no vision, no hearing, maybe no knowledge or ability to recognize in any sense we can understand. Despite Susan's uncomplicated pregnancy, something had gone massively wrong.

I watched over the next several months as Susan and Mandy developed a sort of interdependency, that strange symbiosis that often forms between a special-needs child and her mother. Mandy fed poorly, requiring hours to get a single feeding done. Her twenty-four-hour-a-day needs became Susan's life; there were simply no options. It was a full-time job into which Susan jumped, both physically and emotionally. Very soon, when it came to Mandy and her medical conditions, Susan became the expert. Susan was assertive about her expertise, but never overbearing, and the combination of her crash course in medicine and her mother's intuition resulted in her being right most of the time. If Susan said something had changed with Mandy, you learned to listen up.

At first Susan did what all moms do, she threw herself into an all-out pursuit of the *what* questions. *What* had happened that could have caused her daughter's condition? Just exactly *what* was the full extent of her baby's medical problems? In *what* way did one complicate, compound the other? *What* would the future look like?

The *why* questions remained unanswered but ever present. They seemed to hang in the air at every visit and may actually have been more mine than Susan's. So many patients going through hard times try to answer these *why* questions by turning the hot light on themselves. I think somehow it makes it easier for them. Taking the blame provides some small feeling of control, as if it's easier to believe that they brought this on themselves than to have to face the other two options. That either the world is random and senseless or, sometimes harder yet, that this came into their life at the hands of a loving God. I think Susan wished she could have taken back all the concerns about having a boy; with Mandy's problems I am sure any healthy child would have felt miraculous. But Mandy had apparently worked a kind of magic on her mother because, from the beginning, Susan never seemed to look inside or to doctors or to heaven itself for someone to blame. In the midst of it, Susan had a strong sense of peace about her, a serenity that I have rarely seen. At first I worried about how real it was, concerned that I was watching either a performance or a postponement, that she was burying it all under the legitimate weight of Mandy's medical needs. That was probably more my own projection than anything else. For Susan, I think simply watching what happened to people who came into Mandy's presence day after day was a big part of what kept her going, and it gave at least a partial answer to the why of her daughter's condition.

Our office visits were full of the reports of which of Mandy's specialists had said what and what procedure was being proposed when, etc., etc. My role was complex. I was one part medical translator, one part generalist, one part verifier, one part pastor, and maybe most important of all, I was someone who had touched all the other pieces of this family's life. I knew them in context. I knew their other children. I knew what they did and how they lived before all of this descended upon them. I knew there was more to them than Mandy. The value of this and the therapy it sometimes brings is difficult to grasp. People going through trauma need to know that there is someone who knew them before. Before they were a problem, before the cancer, before they were a victim, before the accident, before the divorce, before the shadow had fallen across their path. Someone who knew that there was more to them than what appeared on their medical problem list. I think the comfort this can bring flows from that tender place inside all of us where we just long to be known. For the Shelleys, weathering the wonder and the storm that was Mandy had a lot to do with being surrounded by a community of friends who continued to walk with them through it.

As the months passed Susan maintained an attitude that spoke both strength and vulnerability. I guess the best word to describe her would be authentic. At some point in every

visit we got down to "How are you doing?" She was honest
in her response. She did not deny what was happening. There
was an enormous cost that came with Mandy, and everybody
paid. Her worries were normal ones. She was concerned that
Mandy would somehow become such a focus that her other
two girls would end up slighted, overlooked. She worried
about her husband, the guy thing—his tendency to hold his
feelings in and the possible consequences of that. We talked
about the plain old physical fatigue of caring for Mandy
24-7. There was no dimension of her family's life that went
unaltered as a result of her youngest daughter. Yet I never
caught her hiding behind any "This is God's will/My cross to
bear" curtain of shallow platitudes. She simply seemed to
accept what was going on for what it was—her life—and she
lived it one day at a time, as really and as best she could.
Susan remained convinced that God brought Mandy into
their lives with a purpose. And she could live without the
whole story of that purpose as long as she had today's edi-
tion. This attitude allowed Susan to embrace both the good
and the bad of it all, maybe suspecting how often the one is
merely a doorway to the other. Day by day, she just kept
going.

Mandy's first year was a kaleidoscope of ever-changing
medical complications. She worked her way through the medical dictionary: strep A, hepatitis B, NG tubes, etc. Three different seizure medications had little impact on her seizures.
There were recurrent pneumonias. Her head stopped growing.
Her neurologic condition deteriorated to the point that she
could not guard her airway during feeding, and a feeding tube
had to be placed. There were frequent respiratory infections

and fevers with obscure causes like suspected urinary tract infections and small pneumonias and multiple hospitalizations and nights at the emergency room. Each storm was weathered for itself, each day accepted with whatever trials and grace it contained. And if any of us did dare to look down the road to that likely day when Mandy would not be with us, we kept it to ourselves until the very end.

When Mandy was almost a year old, Susan became pregnant again. Although there was a lot of murmuring about "how is she possibly going to be able to handle it?" there was a sense of relief in the news. It felt as if there was something to hope for again. There was even more elation when an ultrasound four months into the pregnancy demonstrated this child was a boy. I think there were a few not-so-well-thought-through comments about God "making up for Mandy," which Susan managed to withstand with grace. Although Mandy's care was exhausting and the daily grind of this child's continuous needs was nearly breaking, I don't think Susan ever lost sight of the reality that the rest of us so often either missed or denied. Mandy's time with us, as far as the heart measures it, would not be long enough. And so Susan was able to see beyond the tube feedings and the fevers and the seizures and the constant wondering if something was being missed. Able to see what was the core truth of Mandy's short life—she was, in almost every way that counted, an extreme gift.

It was, however, a short season of hope. A month after learning that the new baby was a boy, Susan was sent for a more sophisticated ultrasound that showed the unthinkable. This child also had multiple birth defects, but unlike with

Mandy, this time the defects were consistent with an already-described syndrome known as trisomy 13. This condition was not in any way related to Mandy's condition, but it left everyone reeling, trying to explain how this could happen to anyone twice. The worst of it was the news that this child's condition was incompatible with life. Most of these children died in utero. If the child were to be born alive, he would die soon afterward. Susan and her husband were wedged between two terrible choices. End it all now or carry the child to term, knowing his likelihood of living even a few minutes was small. Despite the option to end it all with an abortion and the cold quick logic that seemed to come with that, Susan and her husband chose to continue the pregnancy, somehow knowing ahead of time that even minutes with this child would carry lasting value.

I found myself struggling for words throughout the remainder of her pregnancy. I felt like one of Job's friends, obligated in the face of all this to try to explain the ways of God, maybe most of all to myself. And yet, also like Job's friends, I think I was most effective when I just sat and listened. But this was difficult. I felt an overwhelming need to say something, yet in the face of this second tragedy, every word I spoke felt clumsy and crude and wrong. Watching Susan care for Mandy, the whole time knowing that the child she carried had no chance of life, was almost too much to bear. Something inside me wanted to scream at the injustice; something inside me was afraid to get too close. Maybe afraid that if I did, I would draw fire myself.

It felt like I was watching someone take the slow, deliberate, punishing walk to her own personal cross. My position was fixed, and I was left with no choice except to stand there and watch the courage and the cruelty. I saw Susan draw what she needed from several sources. From her own inner strength as a person. From her confidence in a God who loved her. From the friends and family surrounding her. But there was another source I didn't understand at the time. I think God channeled most of the grace Susan needed through Mandy herself. I had gotten it exactly wrong. I had looked at Susan having to care for her needy daughter while carrying a doomed child as falling somewhere between divine mal-practice and a colossally bad cosmic joke. But it was neither. I think more than anything else it was an upside-down kind of grace. Grace standing on its head, to draw our attention, so that even the dullest of us wouldn't miss it. Mandy wasn't Susan's burden. It was she who carried her mother through the dark days until the delivery.

Susan carried her baby almost to term, a small miracle in itself. The delivery was without complication. They named the little boy Toby. Although he lived less than five minutes, those minutes allowed the family to know him and to love him and to grieve him properly.

"When sorrows come they come not single spies, but in battalions." It is very hard to describe what happens to you as the physician in a situation like this, a situation where someone seems to get battered by one tragedy after another. You are left with little to comfort them with except your knowledge that it happens to people with startling regularity. That's probably a small and miserable comfort actually, but true, nonetheless. Certain patients for certain seasons of their lives will seem to act as lightning rods for disaster. You try to imagine what would be the worst possible next thing that could happen to them and *flash,* as soon as your ears stop ringing and the smoke clears, you find your prophecy fulfilled—lightning has struck twice. Every time I saw Susan and Mandy after Toby's death, I thought of how it would have been so much easier if my own personal beliefs did not include the presence of a God who loves. At least I wouldn't have to struggle with the obvious contradiction. But I knew Susan and I shared confidence in a God who knew fully and loved wholly and had the power to make something else happen and yet for some reason, obscure and dark and unsearchable, did not do it.

The focus fell back on Mandy. She continued in and out of the hospital. One infection had brought her close to death about three months before Toby was born. There was a strange occurrence during another of Mandy's hospitalizations. Late one night, as Susan slept, a nurse crept in to check on Mandy. There, hovering above Mandy's hospital crib, was something the nurse could only describe as an angel, moving, floating above her. She could not tell whether the angel was ministering to Mandy or whether it was the other way around. She told Susan this the next morning and Susan, very matter of fact, shared it with me when I came to visit. The most surprising thing about it was how unsurprised we both were. I guess it just seemed natural that Mandy would keep company with angels. It was as if the nurse had simply experienced in a very visual way what most of us who had any contact with Mandy had always known: this world was not Mandy's home.

One of the last times I examined Mandy, I remember

thinking about the paradox of it all. Mandy was flawed and inadequate and helpless in almost every way by which our world measures these things. The list of what she couldn't do and would never do was almost endless. And yet in spite of all the flaws, indeed maybe because of them, she possessed a great power. It was through her wounds that she brought us all together, grew our hearts, and in a way, healed us. And it made me think that once she was gone, it would be through our own wounds that we could continue to do the same for one another. I think that was the music I heard whenever I held her and looked into her eyes. It was Mandy's life message, a message I had unknowingly strained to hear for a long time.

Her last three months of in-and-out-of-the-hospital trips, each more serious than the one before, took their toll. Mandy's general condition never returned to baseline. It was apparent that the slope was now severely downhill. Then came the final hospitalization. Marshall and Susan and I talked extensively about the limits of what we would do. We talked item by item about respirators and resuscitation and medications. Comfort was the key word, and all our measures were to that end. I was surprised by my own reaction. Knowing this day would come didn't make it less difficult. Somehow I thought that with all her problems letting her go would be easier. It wasn't.

I was in my office when the phone call came from the hospital. Mandy had gone into an agonal breathing pattern, implying that death was imminent. I put down the receiver and told my nurse, who turned away and quietly began to weep. I put my hand on her back and tried to comfort her, the whole time wanting someone to comfort me. I canceled the remainder of that afternoon's appointments and drove over to the hospital.

There is something about the death of a child, even a child like Mandy with so many reasons to move on to someplace better, that grips your heart. All you can say is that it is wrong. Without exception, the parents stand engulfed in an unavoidable sea of guilt—the guilt of the survivor, the guilt of having outlived a child and all that feels so unnatural about that. As if a promise has somehow not been kept. A promise each of us whispers into our newborn's ear. A promise to protect, to nourish, to bring to adulthood at least halfway whole and safe and sane.

I was taken aback by the scene that greeted me at the pediatric ward. There were ten or twelve friends who had been called to stand with the Shelleys as they waited for death to come. There were tears mingling with laughter that pretty well mirrored my own internal confusion about what role I was supposed to play. The resuscitation had already stopped.

I embraced Susan and her husband and then went over to Mandy's bed. I listened to Mandy's heart—there was nothing to hear. I checked her widely dilated pupils. I had been drawn by those eyes so many other times. Now I felt a strange longing for the world they once contained. It was as if there had been a wrinkle in the fabric of the universe, and this great soul, momentarily deposited in a limiting little body, had now returned home. As I closed her lids, I felt a sadness sweep over me, a sadness that the gate between our worlds was forever closed. Or at least, closed for now. I then turned to the nurse, marked the time, and pronounced her gone.

Somehow the finality of the statement allowed a torrent of emotion to be loosed in the room. It wasn't a shock or a surprise, it was just final, and until that moment it had never been final. I stepped back and watched the scene, like a player who delivers his short but crucial line, then steps back into the curtains to watch the rest of the play unfold. Susan and her husband embraced first one another and then their friends. They leaned close to Mandy speaking softly, quietly, as if in prayer. I looked down at Mandy's now colorless countenance and was surprised by what I felt at that exact moment. It was out of place, but there was no confusing it— it was jealousy. As I stood there, my mind flashed back to Africa, where my family and I had spent a year volunteering at a missionary hospital outside Nairobi. There was a short-cut to the hospital I used to take every morning that passed through a small missionary graveyard. Now, amid the cacophony of emotions in Mandy's room, I found myself transported to that graveyard, standing in front of one particular stone. The one that captured my heart and imagination the most. It was a small stone pressed flat to the ground with the same birth date and death date carved deeply into it along with one simple phrase:

The first face he saw was Jesus.

Mandy had managed, like that other nameless child, a great magic. She had managed to live among us but, then again, not really among us at all. We all felt sorry for her, as if she had been deprived of so much because of what she would never do, what she would never see. And yet there she lay, and in my heart I knew as surely as I knew anything that when Mandy opened her eyes for the very first time she looked straight into the face of perfection. Her only visual experience would be perfect love, perfect peace, perfect joy. She walked through heaven's gate a pure soul, and I was struck with what a pathetic comedy it was that we pitied her.

Mandy's funeral was a celebration more than anything else. Hers was a good passage; she had known only love if she knew anything at all. I found in the months after her passing that I missed her and thought about her often, and in my dreams she was whole and beautiful and doing everything two-year-olds are supposed to do. I did miss her, but I think what I missed most of all was what happened to me every time she was in the room.

POSTSCRIPT

At Mandy's funeral they released a handful of balloons. First they released a white one, then several pink ones. The white balloon, once released, sped straight up into the sky at a surprising, almost unnatural speed. The pink ones zigzagged slowly up, each taking a different path.

Susan became pregnant within a year of Mandy's death. I think everyone who knew the Shelleys just held their breath. She delivered a perfect, healthy baby boy. They named him Bayly after their good friend Joe Bayly, author of several books, one of which speaks with honesty about what it feels like to lose a child. Bayly is now six years old.

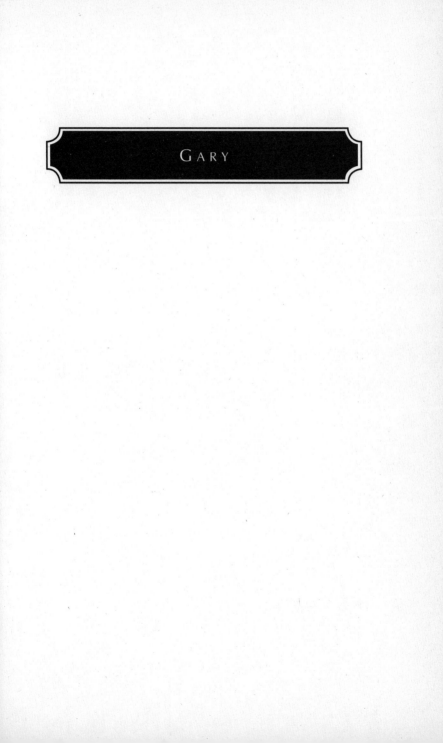

GARY

I was just one more strange request in a day of nothing but strange requests. It started with Mrs. Roberts, one of my "earth mothers," wanting to bring her eight-year-old twins in the room during her pelvic exam. I believe the phrase "educational event" was used. Then it was Renee Morris after that, begging to be fit in right away so we could see her mysterious disappearing rash, which, of course, had mysteriously disappeared by the time she arrived. And now this. Gary Webster had just called and asked my nurse if he could be added as the last patient of the day, and could we meet in my private office rather than an exam room?

"What's up with that?" my nurse asked. When she saw my blank expression, she shook her head and muttered, "There must be something in the water today."

"Yeah, and right about now . . . I wish I had some of it," I shot back. Right before ducking into the next exam room, I shrugged my shoulders and said, "Go ahead and add him."

Gary Webster had been a patient for more than ten years. I had delivered his two boys and knew the family pretty well. He was in his mid thirties, blond, extroverted, and came across a lot like a game-show host. My nurse always referred to him as "Guy Smiley." He had an executive-level job with one of the Christian organizations in town and was also active in the school district—some kind of curriculum committee, leading the conservative charge. He was affable and outgoing and friendly but seemed to fly at one fixed altitude. No matter what the relationship, Gary was Gary. Whether you knew him for five minutes or fifteen years, you got pretty much the same thing. I was never quite sure whether there just wasn't much more there or if he was intentionally keeping people at arm's distance. I chalked it up to a guy thing.

Before I went in to see my last regular patient of the day, my nurse said, "I just put Mr. Webster upstairs in your office. Do you think you'll need me?" She was giving me that "please say no, please say no, please say no" look.

"No, go ahead and go home after this patient," I said and smiled. "If I need anything, I'll call one of the evening nurses. Thanks."

When I finished with my last patient, I went up to my private office on the second floor. I rarely used this office for patient visits. It was out of the way, and I reserved it mostly for paperwork, quiet moments, and the delivery of bad news. I walked in and found Gary sitting on the small couch on the wall across from my desk. Above the couch was a large painting of a shepherd leading a flock of sheep up to higher pasture. On the opposite wall were twelve eight-by-ten pictures of our daughters that my wife had put together. Gary took the initiative, got up, and shook my hand right away. I couldn't help but feel he was always campaigning.

"Hey, great pictures of your kids. Thanks so much for seeing me like this. I'm sorry to make you stay late." He always seemed to be booming, as if he were addressing a crowd without the benefit of a mike. "You know, I don't even know if you're the one I should be talking to. I just needed to talk to someone about this and, Jim, you were the one who kept coming to mind." I was vaguely irritated by his use of my first name.

I took off my white coat, hung it on the hook by the door, pulled a chair closer to the couch, and sat down. "That's fine, Gary. If I'm not the one, then maybe I can help steer you toward someone who is. What's going on? How can I help?" I was tuning in my happy Dr. Judge "I've got all the time in the world" thing. What I really hoped was that this would be short and simple. It had been a long day and I wanted to go home.

Gary sat on the couch, bent forward, his legs spread widely apart, elbows resting on his knees; as if he were in a huddle, getting ready to discuss the next play. One hand held the other, the thumb of his left hand rubbing repeatedly over the same place on the base of his right thumb, trying to rub off some spot that only he could see. Once he got started, he looked mostly at the floor or out the window toward the park across the street. His looks at me felt timed, coinciding with particular points in his story where he needed to get some read on my reaction. Most patients come into the office, sure that their story is the most shocking one you have ever heard. Little do they know. A rotation or two through the ER and pretty soon most doctors are convinced that just about nothing could surprise them anymore. Gary certainly tested that assumption. He turned the volume down on his voice.

"What I'm going to tell you is just between us, right? I

wouldn't want you to even tell Jan, although she pretty well knows everything already."

I studied him there on the couch. He was nervous, setting up the rules, and he didn't want me saying anything to his wife, who supposedly knew "everything already." By this point in our conversation I was already sure of where we were headed. There is only one subject that brings men in with this kind of urgency and this kind of awkwardness. Whatever was bothering Gary had something to do with sex.

"Gary, whatever we talk about is always confidential. I wouldn't talk to anyone about this without your permission . . ." Speech 103—patient confidentiality.

"And I wouldn't want any of this written down, either," he continued. "You never know who is going to get a hold of your medical record."

Speech 106—ethical issues regarding patient records. " . . . so don't worry about that, Gary. Whatever I put in your chart will be very obscure and vague. It will probably say something like 'Discussed personal concerns.' That's it. You can look at it any time you want."

"Personal concerns." He forced a short, nervous laugh, oozing self-derision. "Yeah, that about sums it up."

He looked at me long and hard. Like that moment when you're standing on the high dive, wondering if you have it in you to jump. You're momentarily suspended between two nearly equal forces—one drawing you back, one pulling you forward. Safety and cowardice lie behind you, fear and bravery in front. Will you do it? Gary blinked a couple times, swallowed, then took the plunge.

"It's all about pornography, Jim. I think I've got this

problem with pornography." He waited a few seconds, then went on. "No, no check that. I know I've got a problem. A big problem."

As he said it, I could feel him scanning me, searching for any trace of reaction. Judgment? Horror? Sympathy? Forgiveness? I'm not sure what I was feeling at the time. Did it matter anyway? What I was sure of was that the empathetic "tell me all about it" look was even now flooding my face. After ten years in practice, it had become reflexive, a part of the job. I couldn't have stopped it if I'd wanted to. Every day, I felt less and less of the distance between that look and whatever it was I actually felt inside.

"Tell me about it, Gary. What kind of problem are we talking about here? How did it get started?" Let the confession begin.

Something in my face or the setting or his own overwhelming need opened the door just a little bit and allowed the story to come rushing out. Or at least part of it. It was an old story.

"You know I travel with my job. I travel a lot. You remember, I barely made it back from a trip for our youngest, Danny's, birth."

I didn't remember, of course, because that had been eight years and about a hundred deliveries ago. But for each patient it was a singular momentous event, and each is convinced that the doctor must remember it all as well as they do. I shook my head, meaning "go on," knowing that he would interpret it to mean I remembered. Hopefully a forgivable insincerity.

"I don't know what made me do it the first time. I wasn't into it in any big way in college." He looked down at his hand. "Who knows?" He thought a minute, then said, "You know, I think the truth was I was just bored and a little bit lonely. Jan and I have always had a good sex life. I love her; I really do." His eyes got moist as he continued. "But I was just sitting there all alone in this hotel room at night, and there was nothing on TV, and before I knew it I was reading through the titles on the adult movie channel. I was curious. I thought I'd just check it out is all. I only watched about half of the movie, then got to feeling so guilty I turned it off. But I couldn't get the images out of my head. For the next couple of days, it was like, like that movie just kept playing." He stopped and looked over at me. I think he was trying to assess whether or not it was safe to keep going.

There's an old joke that goes like this:

Q: How do you know your life is really, really boring?
A: When the priest interrupts your confession to ask you if you know a seven-letter word for an African blackbird.

Now, I wasn't exactly doing crossword puzzles in my head at this point, but for sure, this was definitely not a new story. Maybe I was just becoming a little numb to it all. Although each patient's story had its own unique elements and end points, the structure of the story and the themes were often consistent. It was all about getting caught up in something that, in the end, catches you. The beginnings, like his, were often small and inconsequential. I had yet to run into anyone who'd stumbled once, then plunged headlong into their own personal hell. Most of the time they arrived there standing up, having taken a long and lazy winding road with a very subtle slope. I suppose there is a kind of strategy to it. No one seems to notice the rate of descent. No one gets a good hard look at what's waiting for them up ahead.

Gary went on, his courage apparently bolstered by the fact that uttering the words had not caused flaming hail to rain down upon us. "Before I knew it, watching the adult movie channel was a regular feature of every business trip. Each time, I went through the same stupid sequence. I'd think about it ahead of time, look forward to it, anticipate it. Before long I was planning my trips around it. I would pur- posely avoid scheduling anything with anyone in the evenings so I could sit in the hotel room and get off watching the movie. It was like my reward or something. Then afterward, the same awful guilt. Can you imagine? Here I was talking all day about church business, and at night I'm sitting in some hotel room watching stuff I'm embarrassed to even describe. Every time, every time I promised myself it was the last time, that tomorrow would be different. But it never was. I just kept at it, over and over again." Almost as an afterthought he added, "That was nearly ten years ago."

Gary's head was down, and he was shaking it back and forth, wiping away tears almost before they appeared. He con- tinued with more examples of his entanglement with pornog- raphy. There was a steady increase in the scope of the problem: the Internet, cable channels, adult video houses. His descriptions were more detailed and graphic than necessary, but part of what he needed was to be able to put words to what he was entangled in. For me, the primary shock value of the story was in how long it had gone on. I remember thinking

THE CLOSEST OF STRANGERS

at the time of a line from the novel *Lady Chatterley's Lover* we had been forced to memorize years ago in senior English. The main character is asked by a friend how she could have kept up her repeated infidelities. Her reply seemed to describe Gary's situation. "At first I thought that I would die of shame, but then . . . shame died."

The other reason I think I was taking this all in stride was that I had just completed a lot of reading regarding addictive behavior in preparation for a radio interview about the subject. Gary was telling a classic addiction story. The slow and seemingly innocent beginning, the rapid acceleration, the controlling insanity of it all, the endless treadmill of excitement and guilt and remorse and fixation and doing it all over again. Addictive behavior is, more than anything else, a cold compress on a bad wound. It's a crude attempt to fill a void it can never satisfy, a void that only enlarges with each accommodation. Patients forever try to fill that void with something. You name it: alcohol or drugs or gambling or pornography or food or shopping or sex. Whatever momentary satisfaction they achieve only leaves them guilt-ridden and hungry for more. It is an endless whirlpool of diminishing returns, sucking the person in deeper and faster until they are eventually dragged to the bottom. Each person has his or her own personal tolerance, but eventually everyone cries out for help in one way or another. And often it's the family doctor who gets the first call. I knew one thing for sure. When you heard it, you needed to act fast because someone caught in an addiction finds hope as hard to hold on to as reality.

I started into my addictive behavior speech. "Gary, you're describing more than just dabbling with a little pornography.

You're describing what sounds like something out of your control over a long period of time. I know it sounds strange but . . . this could be an addiction." Now it was my turn to do the scanning, and I could sense his shields going up. "Gary, people can get addicted to lots of things other than drugs and alcohol. Whenever anything, substance or behavior, starts to dominate your life, you're dealing with a possible addiction. I don't think I'm overreacting here. I've seen this sequence too many times and I'll tell you, it can carry serious consequences for you, your marriage, your whole life." He was focused on me with what felt like practiced sincerity. Like a high school football player more worried about convincing his coach he's listening, than listening itself. "Be careful. It's easy to tell yourself that it's no big deal. Frankly, I think you've probably been telling yourself that for years. Trying to rationalize it away and convince yourself that it's not really hurting any-one, that you can stop it any time, but that's a lie. It is hurt-ing someone, most particularly you. And if you can stop it, then why haven't you?" Something hit with the last couple of sentences. I could see him start to soften up a little. I slowed my words. "There's a broken record here that keeps playing over and over again—fixation, obsession, followed by repeat-ing the behavior in the same way over and over again. Then the sexual release followed by guilt and despair. Gary, these are the features of every addiction."

Gary's expression had become almost grave, and there was a cloud of anxiety darkening his gray eyes. He was strug-gling. It was as if he knew he was drowning and he wanted to grab hold of the lifesaver, but there was something he was afraid of. I couldn't tell whether he was afraid he didn't have the strength to hold on or afraid he really didn't want to get out of the water.

I got up, walked over to my desk, and started fishing around in the top drawer. I'd played my part, time for a little player substitution. "Gary, I'm going to give you a card with the address and phone number of a psychologist I know." He flinched immediately. "Now, don't worry. This doesn't mean I think you're crazy. It just means that this is a battle that needs to be fought on all fronts at the same time. There's a medical aspect and an emotional aspect and a spiritual aspect. We have to hit all three."

His face tightened up right away and he interrupted, almost frantic.

"It can't be anyone in town, Jim. You know what it's like: something like this gets out and I'm out of a job in about ten seconds." Again a bitter little half-laugh. "The Christian community can be anything but Christian when it comes to this kind of thing." He drew a deep breath, shook his head, and looked up at the ceiling. "You have no idea. You don't know how many times I've begged God to take this away, but it just keeps happening. All I'm getting is silence. I wanted to tell my pastor, tell someone, but c'mon, this isn't the kind of thing people talk about in church."

I felt a sadness sweep over me as I realized he was right. When it came to sin, there seemed to be an ecclesiastical gentleman's agreement: no specifics, please; keep it generic. Which only leaves people to draw their own false conclusions. They're struggling with problems that aren't generic, problems with dirty brand names like adultery and pornography, convinced that the worst thing anyone else struggles with is putting the shopping carts back in their rack at the grocery store. A church that had the courage to help people battling addictive behavior was a rare find. I looked at him and thought of the bitter irony of it all. Sunday after Sunday there Gary sat, probably in the same pew, with men who struggled in the same way he did, some winning some losing, each doomed to live out their struggle in sanitary isolation. Each one immobilized by the fear that he was the only one. I thought of the miracles that might result if just one of them would stand up and tell his story. But that was unlikely to happen. Not with everyone else looking so perfect and problem-free. If a church was intended to be anything, it seemed to me, it was intended to be a community of healing. But healing can't begin until we drop the pretense that no one's wounded.

"I know what you mean, Gary." I handed him the card. "This is someone out of the area. I think you'll feel safe there, and I think you'll be able to talk freely." We shook hands; he thanked me. I asked him to come back in two weeks and then showed him the way out. As I sat back down at my desk to finish up my paperwork, I couldn't get the encounter out of my head. The scenes he'd described and my own feelings were swirling around inside, but didn't feel attached. Why was I feeling so uneasy? Was it his heavy penance? It did seem a little out of proportion. Maybe I was just getting callous to it all. Was it his concern about keeping it secret? Secrets have power, extreme power that can feed the addiction. Or was it simply how alone he seemed? I tried to shake it off and finally went home.

I received a courtesy call from the psychologist I sent

him to about three days later. Gary had called the same evening I'd seen him to set up an appointment. The psychologist agreed this was definitely an addiction, and he scheduled regular weekly visits for a while. He had also recommended a sexual addictions group that was specifically designed for people with a Christian background. Gary was very iffy about this. There was a short silence on the phone before the psychologist added, "From what he's telling me, it's gone on a long time at one level. That's unusual for addictions . . . I'll keep you posted."

Two weeks later I met Gary again in my private office to follow up, once again the last patient of the day. It was awkward at first. I think when a patient shares something like he had, there is an anxiety that plagues them soon afterward. It's a feeling of vulnerability, made proportionally more intense by the physician's invulnerability. Inevitably, the questions start. "Should I have done it? Can he really be trusted with what I told him? What does he think of me now?" In any other setting, intimacy on this level is earned with time and trust and mutuality. But in a doctor's office the "MD" alone is supposed to justify it. Sometimes the letters just aren't enough.

I don't know if it was my imagination or not, but there seemed to be a little less of "Guy Smiley" this time. Gary spoke at a normal volume. Unusual for him. "Thanks for the referral, Jim. I really feel like I can talk to that guy. He makes it easy." He drew a deep breath. "He agrees with you; he thinks I've got an addiction going on here." Then he added, "I went to my first group meeting a couple days ago." He rolled his eyes. "Whew, that was weird. I didn't say very much, just sort of hung out in the back and watched. At least it's nice to know I'm not the only one who's screwed up." He looked at me expectantly. Expecting what, I didn't know.

"Gary, the important thing is that you're getting help. That's what counts." As I said the words, it struck me how meaningless, banal, and detached they sounded. It felt like I'd just thrown him a bone. It wasn't what I wanted to say. I think what I wanted to say was something about how we are all screwed up, about how his story had touched me, made me think about my own isolation. I wanted to defend people in self-help groups as at least having some vague inkling of what was going on inside them. At least they were beyond pretending they didn't have a problem. But there was a voice in my head telling me to shut up and stay professional. It was a voice I had gotten used to listening to.

"Yeah, well, you're probably right." I don't know whether Gary missed my superficiality or forgave it. He hurried into the rest of his report. "Anyway, one of the things we're supposed to do with this Twelve Step thing is to meet regularly with someone and come clean about what's going on. Someone other than yourself and God." He said it with a juvenile kind of singsong to his voice, as if it were some silly homework assignment he was obligated to complete. I didn't think that was how he really felt. I think he was protecting himself against rejection, setting up a possible "exit with dignity" strategy in case he didn't get a positive response.

"And anyway, seeing as how you know a lot of the story already, I was thinking of maybe asking you to be that person." He was pretending to be casual, but there was a readable intensity to his eyes.

Now, this caused a weird reaction in me. In one way I was

flattered. It indicated a lot of trust on his part, or at least a sense that I was the safest person he could ask. But in another way it scared me. It didn't feel safe, and I had made a professional lifestyle out of staying safe. The mix of the implied mutuality and the quasi-medical nature of the problem made me insecure.

"It's really almost more the role of a friend than a doctor," I said, half joking, half serious. I think I was looking for a way out.

He looked at me and for a moment dropped his guard entirely, and said as openly as I had ever heard him say anything, "I guess what I'm saying is, right now . . . I need both."

With this began a series of Wednesday appointments. Always the same time, five-thirty, always in my private office, always the last patient of the day. Over the next several weeks Gary forged into the uncharted territory of telling the truth about himself. And as for me, I smiled and encouraged and tried to say the right thing, but continued to hide behind the starched safety of my white coat. It was no longer patient and doctor; it was just as much teacher and student. Only this time I was the student. I watched with jealous interest as he began to speak honestly about himself. About what he lacked and what his strengths were, of how he was unraveling the mystery of how years of deception had neutered his faith. He taught me more about what it is to be entangled in an addiction than I wanted to know. He described the constant tension that had become part of his every day. Over the years the life-and-death combat between the angel and the ape that resided inside consumed him, transformed him, reduced him. More and more of his emotional energy was being sucked into the addiction. Thinking about it, regretting it, protecting it, loving it, hating it. As more life flowed into the addiction, it seemed to drain out of everything else. He found himself trading realities. The world of his addiction became more real while the world of his family and faith and job faded into life-less routine. He felt like he was running from shadow to shadow, sentenced to perpetual hiding, and the hiding had turned him into a caricature of himself. It was this aspect of his story I couldn't seem to let go of.

About two months into it Gary came into my office more on edge than usual. He looked nervous and jittery. As I took the chair opposite him, it was apparent this session was going somewhere else.

He seemed to rush at me with his words. "Jim, there's more I need to tell you about." He waited, looked out the window, then fixed me in his sight, his face full of fear and insistence. "If I don't . . ." He swallowed hard. "If I don't, then these meetings are really just a joke. I have to be able to be honest with someone. Get it all out on the table." He was breathing heavily and rocking as he spoke, maybe trying to comfort himself. He finally settled into that same huddle-up position he had taken the first time we met.

"It's okay, Gary. You know you can tell me anything. That's what this is supposed to be all about. You've been pretty honest already." I was experiencing a serious dis-connect between my words and my feelings right then. I really did not want to hear any more.

"Honest? Not honest enough. That's for sure. There's a lot I left out." I thought I had heard enough details already, but it was apparent he wasn't going to hold back. I felt myself tense as he plowed ahead. "The pornography sets the stage for wanting to play it all out in reality. After watching it a hundred or so times, you start to convince yourself that acting it out wouldn't be that much worse." He was pushing his words, as if he was afraid that if he even stopped for a breath he would lose his momentum and not be able to continue.

"It happened the first time when Jan and the boys were out of town. I think they were visiting her mother. Somehow their being away gave me some kind of excuse. I don't know, I think knowing I wouldn't have to face them right away made doing it easier." He started rocking again. "I went up to this adult bookstore to get a movie and ended up spending about an hour there. I was pretending to look for a movie, but I was really looking for something more. I don't know why, but in some sick way I always felt comfortable there, like . . . like I wasn't alone or something. There was every conceivable kind of person there. Guys in suits and derelicts and working guys and students." As he went on, it started to feel like he was no longer talking to me. He was looking through me, past me, as if the words were for someone else. The speed of his speech accelerated, like a train hurtling out of control.

" . . . and just, just being there somehow made me feel relaxed. Like, like we were all just a bunch of naughty little boys. Next thing you know I'm talking to some guy, and he's telling me where I can go for some real action . . . or maybe I asked him." At this point he started to cry, but he kept on, not seeming to notice his own tears. "There's a whole parallel world, Jim, going on right beside this one." The volume and the octave of his voice both jumped a level. "Massage parlors, strip clubs, and worse. You pay for it and you can get anything. The first time, it . . . it felt dangerous just to be there. It was like a huge adrenaline rush. It was like a fix. I . . . I . . . I started going to those places, going real regular and . . . pretty soon it's like a ritual. Every time, I needed more and more."

By this time he was visibly trembling, as if he were going to explode. He went down on one knee, sobbing, his shoulders shaking.

I gripped the arms of my chair. Inside I felt a thick cloud of emotion that was obscure and faceless. I felt like I was supposed to say something, anything. But I couldn't speak. It was like that moment in a bad dream when you stand there paralyzed, screaming as hard as you can, but you can't make any sound. I sat there mute and wordless. Maybe it was only me who felt the unformed words choking in my throat. Gary kept going, proceeding through a full confession that detailed a hidden life of ritualized anonymous sexual contacts that contradicted his known life in almost every way.

Despite what he was talking about, or maybe because of it, there was almost a holiness to the moment. I knew he was uttering something of the dark essence of who he was, defenseless and naked and vulnerable. In the confession of all his broken promises was buried a greater confession. It was the confession of his own brokenness. Of the fact that he could not put this back together himself. It was a place he had to get to, a place where he could finally turn around and return home. He had wandered in the "far country" long enough.

His confession was the final act that moved him beyond

regret to repentance. Until now, I think he had only regretted what he had done. The stupidity and the waste and the widening gap between people's perceptions and who he knew himself to be. He regretted it all. I'd seen plenty of regret in my career, and the emotion that always seemed to infuse it was anger. Anger at yourself or others. Anger over something precious that was lost. But as I looked at Gary, I saw very little anger. The emotion that hung heavy in the room was something very different—it was fear, a choking fear. Fear, because I think, at its core, repentance is turning around, burning a bridge, giving something up, leaving something behind. Something that was hated and cherished at the same time. The addiction had at least temporarily eased some deep, black, and nameless pain inside him. Now what? What confidence did he have that it would ever be filled? And so he was afraid.

As I listened to him, I felt a certain resonance inside, and it made me wonder whether close to the epicenter of all our souls lies a confession like his, a confession about the true state of our souls and what it is we lack. A confession that until uttered holds us wordless, without any way of speaking, really speaking, to God or ourselves or to those around us. I watched full of jealousy and wonder as Gary, between sobs and tears, began to speak a new language, a strange, honest language with a harsh beauty to it that made me long to be able to speak it myself. He made his complete confession, and I listened and said nothing, imprisoned in my chair, bound by my white coat. Answerless. I'd like to think my silence in some way hallowed the moment. I don't know, maybe that's wishful thinking. All I know is that as the moment passed, it became clear to me who was on the road to healing and who wasn't.

We tested Gary for HIV and looked for other evidence of venereal disease. Miraculously, despite years of this activity and scores of nameless sexual contacts, all the tests were negative. What I witnessed that day in the office was a beginning. Life began to flow in the opposite direction, away from the addiction, which he still struggled with, and toward his counseling and his faith and his marriage. Whatever wall he had put up dividing himself from the other people in his addictions group came down. As the months passed, the most powerful of the healing forces at work in his life was his faith. He began to work through the questions that had dogged him for the last ten years.

Later he told me, "You know what, Jim? All those years, I kept accusing God of not helping me. Of leaving me. Of not listening to me. Why didn't he step in and pull me out of this?" Clear-eyed and sincerely he looked at me and said, "I think I had to get to a point where I could admit to myself that the reason he was distant was because I had moved, not him. He wasn't going to make me give it up; I had to come to a point where I was willing to do that." Gary never said God took the addiction away, but he became more and more confident that together they could overcome it. Months later he told me it was his faith that empowered his recovery. It empowers it still.

He told his wife, Jan, the whole story the same night he told me. She was devastated. She knew something was going on but had no idea of the enormity of the problem. She had spent years standing by helplessly as her husband slowly faded out. The frustration and anger made me wonder if they would make it. But somehow, she reached down inside and found the strength and the grace to forgive him and, more than this, to stand with him. They began a serious rebuilding process, and their marriage seemed to take on a new reality. She was badly wounded and confused by all the deception and infidelity, but she never let go of a bedrock confidence that their marriage was intended to last. She held on.

After several months my meetings with Gary became less frequent and eventually just stopped happening. Frankly, I wasn't all that sorry to see it end. I think I felt a little used. Maybe that was my own fault, the price of keeping it so professional. It's easy to forget what a blessing it is to be naive, easy to forget that listening can be costly. You aren't a machine that can erase the tape at will. The patient's file may stay on your desk, but what they have told you becomes a part of your own permanent record. I was left with the knowledge of a world I didn't want to know about.

Patients have their own reasons for eventually not wanting to come back. Over time, I think, there is almost a resentment that builds up. The doctor becomes synonymous with the disease, a living symbol of the problem, of a troubled place in a patient's life from which he or she has moved on. No one wants to be reminded any more frequently than they have to about their darkest moments. There is also something deadly about the one-sided nature of confession. It carries with it a "holier than thou, you're wounded, I'm not" implication. In Gary's case, I certainly hadn't done anything to contradict that idea. But maybe, most of all, it's the simple fact that you are someone who knows their secret. And each time they look at you, they know they are looking into the full face of their confessor. Confession needs to be followed by absolution, but absolution is not ours to grant. I think I know now why there is a screen in the confessional. In the end, it protects both priest and penitent.

POSTSCRIPT

Two years later Gary took a new job and moved away. It must have given him the feeling of a fresh start. He took a position that required no traveling, and I think with that decision he built a kind of protective hedge around his new life. I haven't heard from him for several years.

One evening, months after I had stopped seeing Gary regularly, I was sitting at my desk doing charts. I looked up at the painting above the couch, the one of the shepherd leading the flock of sheep, and started thinking about Gary. Why was I still so unsettled by the whole episode? Almost resentful. Maybe it was because it forced me to look at myself. Years of vicarious emotional living had reduced me to my own caricature. I had become emotionally mute, and my wordlessness was seeping from the office into the rest my life. I was haunted by the moment when Gary finally broke down and I couldn't speak, couldn't identify what I was feeling, let alone express it. It was a metaphor for what I had become. I looked at the painting again, then picked up the phone and called a counselor. It was time for the doctor to become the patient.

JULIE

At first glance her life appeared to be pretty much perfect. Perhaps, a little too perfect. That probably should have been my first clue. Julie could have been a poster child for the good life. She was a walking commercial: the end result of a lot of right choices, starting with the right toothpaste and working her way up to the right perfume, the right cereal, the right clothes, the right car, the right home, the right husband. From all outward appearances, Julie had definitely arrived. But whenever I saw her in the office, I couldn't shake the feeling that I was watching a performance. Maybe it was the vague scripted quality to so much about her. Maybe it was the way she kept sneaking glances at herself in the mirror on the wall beside her as we talked. Maybe it was the too-deliberate nature of her entrances and exits. It felt like *The Truman Show* in reverse, as if her life was a moment-by-moment on-screen event, but instead of the whole world watching, Julie was the only one tuning in. She seemed stuck on stage, searching for the best camera angle, always just a little bit tense. Afraid, maybe most of all, that someone would start to ad-lib.

She was beautiful in a Waspy, white-bread kind of way,

petite and pushing the envelope on thin. But there was an edge to Julie's perfection, something harsh, almost mechanical that drew you in then pushed you quickly away. The edge served a purpose. It insured that no one would get any closer than she intended, certainly not close enough to get a good look at her without the makeup and the lights. There was another odd thing about her perfection. The combination of it all—the perfect face and perfect hair and perfect clothes and perfect world—when blended together, yielded something rather imperfect. Something bland and flat and almost mannequin-like. Something, in the final analysis, perfectly forgettable.

Julie was a corporate wife in her mid thirties. Our suburb is one of four or five Chicago suburbs where a lot of corporate people tend to land. They are viewed with a degree of suspicion by the local townies, who I think see them more as modern nomads who don't belong to Middle America, nomads who are just passing through. "Corporates" are looked upon as a distinct subculture, for whom a series of values, or maybe more to the point, nonvalues, immediately apply. All that moving around tells you something about what they don't value: things like relationships or stability or laying down roots. One thing they do appear to value is their own image and all the necessary hand mirrors that go along with it, like money and career and conspicuous consumption. From the locals' perspective, the corporates' greatest crime boils down to one thing—they don't put family first.

And in this particular suburb, that falls pretty high up on The Top Ten List of Unforgivable Sins, somewhere between racial intolerance and failing to recycle.

Julie's husband, Cameron, was an ex–college football player who had parlayed his easy all-American charm, good looks, and competitive spirit into a successful investment banking career. Money had come very easily, but I think he was experiencing at midlife a certain truth: wealth without work can extract a high price, often payable only in the currency of your own soul. Now coming up fast on forty, he found himself encountering a nondescript restlessness. Work, his investments, and his family were all running on cruise control. The easy achievement of his goals, living a commercial-perfect life, had left him without a sense of winning. And he seemed acutely aware that the clock was ticking. He had that look men often get when they start searching for something new to fill the growing hollowness inside, a void all the more powerful because it has no name.

I usually saw Cameron once a year for his annual "do everything whether I need it or not" corporate physical. His examination was always a bit humorous. Despite the fact he was in perfect physical condition, he could not seem to relax. He approached it like some kind of entrance exam and stayed on the defensive throughout the entire encounter. To him, my standard questions were tantamount to an interrogation behind enemy lines. Anything besides name, rank, and serial number was information that could be used against him. It was almost as if he was convinced that if he answered yes to any of the "ever have" questions, even the ones everyone answers yes to—like headaches or back pain or stomach symptoms—he would be fined. I think he saw it all as some kind of high-stakes game, where the penalty for losing is a forced admission of your own mortality. Maybe what he feared more than anything was the quickly approaching "someday soon" when his charm and good looks would no longer be enough.

As far as I could see, Julie's relationship with her husband was what would best be described as functional. They functioned well together and played complementary roles. He provided her with the lifestyle she had decided early on she intended to become accustomed to. She in turn gave him what he wanted, a virtual Stepford wife. She was pretty to look at, made their home a showcase, and was always agreeable, never complaining about his travel or moving when the almighty career called. But something about them haunted me with its absence. There was a profound lack of warmth, or any emotionality for that matter, on both their parts. In the four years I knew them, I can't remember actually seeing them in the same room together. It was as if they worked for the same company, just on different shifts.

Julie consistently talked about Cameron in the third person, rarely calling him by name.

"My husband's out of town right now but will be back sometime Thursday. I'll tell him to call your office about his results." Or, "My husband wants me to find out what we can do to stop these ear infections. He thinks the children are sick way too often."

It struck me that from her description he could easily have been someone she knew a lot about, but hadn't actually met. As for Cameron, if I had to rely on what he told me, I'm not sure I would have known he even had a wife and family.

Yet it all looked pretty good on the outside, as long as you didn't probe too deeply and only viewed them from just the right angle. What things looked like to others seemed to be pretty much the name of their game. Image maintenance was Julie's full-time occupation, and it was obvious she had had a lot of practice. But there were some cracks beginning to show through. Small ones at first. For instance, Julie was in my office much more often than other patients, always in the name of the children's health. Her "he just doesn't look right to me" visits were averaging about twice a month per child, which meant I was seeing her for some reason almost once a week. I'd certainly seen this pattern before. Sometimes it's simply a case of mistaken identity, a muted, garbled cry for help on the part of the mother, trying to push itself to the surface. Unwilling or unable to identify themselves as the needy one, some moms keep bringing their children into the office, subconsciously hoping someone will recognize them as the true patient.

During these visits, from time to time, I would catch a glimpse of a different Julie. It always came the same way, a fleeting moment when the mask seemed to slip just a bit, always while half looking the other way. I thought at first it was inadvertent, but now I'm not so sure. Now I wonder if those moments were not a trail of bread crumbs left by Julie herself. I saw in her a certain searching quality that had a strong sense of déjà vu. It was as if she were lost in a giant hall of mirrors, groping for a way out, unsure of where image left off and reality began. I knew only too well what that felt like. The more I got to know her, the sadder it made me feel, because I knew that somewhere buried beneath all the lacquered layers of expectations was a real person. I wondered what it would take to dig her out from under the weight of it all. I wondered if, in fact, she even wanted to be rescued.

Perfection, even when it's only skin deep, is hard to maintain. It takes a lot of energy and I've never seen anyone keep it up forever. Julie eventually found that out.

Several months passed during which I didn't see Julie or her children. I wondered whether they had moved or if I had offended them somehow. I even checked their charts to see if one of my partners had seen them. Then one day I saw Julie's name, not her kids, on my schedule of appointments. The reason listed for the visit was "check tiredness." When I walked into the exam room, I had to take a second look because I almost didn't recognize her. The makeup was barely there, the hair was less than perfect, and she was wearing a wrinkled sweat suit. Her battery was apparently starting to run down.

She began with some defensive posturing right away.

"Well, I think it's just the flu, really, but my husband told me I had to get this checked out." The way she said it didn't reflect much personal concern on Cameron's part. It was more like getting her "checked out" came third on his to-do list, right after getting the oil changed in the Jaguar and calling the gardener.

"I just feel so tired lately; I have absolutely no energy. Just getting out of bed in the morning's a chore," she said, sighing deeply, looking as if for the first time in a long time she wasn't working off a script.

"Tired and no energy" translates into a great deal of time and testing in order to arrive at a diagnosis. It is made even more difficult by the knowledge that the vast majority of people with these complaints have very little purely physical going on. Doctors, most particularly primary-care doctors, have to make a decision early on in their professional lives. Stress and depression put on a myriad of different faces. Maybe as much as 50 percent of what a doctor sees every day has an emotional base. If a doctor decides his job is merely weeding out the 50 percent that is not emotionally rooted and letting the rest fend for itself, I think he or she is left with the question, Have I really done my job? Pain is pain, whether it comes at the hand of a lot of wrong choices or bacteria. No matter what the cause of a person's problem or pain a doctor has made a promise to help. This promise means using all the tools in your arsenal, including the thera-peutic tool most often overlooked—yourself. Because it's people you're dealing with day in and day out, sometimes it's not as a physician that you bring the greatest therapy. Some-times it's as a fellow struggler. A fellow struggler who by lis-tening and sharing a little of his own life can at times go way beyond the boundaries of antibiotics and procedures.

And so I began by listening, listening actively, and giving Julie permission to talk about things she was not accustomed to talking about.

"Julie, as you might expect, feeling tired and having no energy can have about a thousand causes that range any-where from cancer to depression," I began. It's important to say the words out loud because it's the unsaid words that have the most power and seem to cause the most damage. So right from the start I've learned to give a voice to the patient's worst fears. You certainly aren't going to come up with any-thing they haven't already lain in bed at night worrying about. Anyone who suddenly begins feeling grossly tired and isn't thinking about cancer or brain tumors or something worse has either not watched enough soaps or not shared these symptoms with their mother. When something suddenly changes, I think we all begin a deadly game of "fill in the blank," and an accelerating dialogue is put into motion. "This time it could be cancer, it could be MS; it could be painful, it could be judgment for something I did; it could be unfair. This time . . . it could be me." And marching right alongside each "could be" is a specific fate. But as you are dragged along in this parade, trying to reconcile yourself to the twenty or so worst-case scenarios, you discover a certain truth. The grace to get by does not apply to the "could be's." It only works on "what is."

And so I began the long and tedious job of unraveling: a process every bit as delicate, every bit as important, requiring every bit as much skill and finesse as a surgical procedure. The problem is insurance and managed-care companies don't quite see it that way. It's hard to get reimbursed for listening. The pressure put on physicians to see more patients in less time is self-defeating because it pushes doctors to substitute expensive and ever-expanding medical technology for the simple act of listening. Julie didn't need a CAT scan or two thousand dollars' worth of blood work. She needed someone to take the time, ask the right questions, and hear what she was saying.

"Tell me about your sleep pattern, Julie. Has it changed at all?"

"Yes, for sure," she replied. "It's weird. I get to sleep okay, I guess. In fact I'm so tired I just seem to melt the minute I get the kids into bed around 9:30. But almost every night I wake up sometime between two and four and just lie there staring at the ceiling, wide awake, the whole world trooping through my head. It's so frustrating. I can't seem to get back to sleep no matter what. I toss and turn till about five in the morning when I end up dropping off to sleep again, only to have to get up by 6:30 to get the kids going. Then when I wake up I feel like I've been drugged."

I could see a pattern starting to emerge. "And what about your appetite? Any changes there? Anything happening with your weight?"

"My appetite is down, way down. I'm just not interested in eating," Julie continued. She was beginning to relax a little, letting her guard down just a bit. "I think I've lost about five or six pounds without even trying." She paused a moment then added, "It's scaring me."

"Any other changes you've noticed, Julie? In your activities, in your exercise, outside involvements? Attitude toward sex?" I asked.

"No, not really. I'm still doing most of the same stuff I've always done. What choice do I have? But it's an effort. Everything's an effort. Getting out of bed in the morning's an effort; making the kid's lunches is an effort. I can't even think about exercise."

I didn't let it go. "And sex, any changes there?"

Julie drew a deep breath and looked at me with a look that had flashes of pain and vulnerability and a little hostility. She lowered her voice and slowed the cadence of her words, like when you're sharing a secret.

"Dr. Judge, my husband and I . . . we only have sex about

twice a year. Makes it kinda hard to see any change." She followed it with a bitter little laugh. I think she read something on my face. Then she added, "Oh, that's just fine from my perspective. I don't know what he does about it." Her voice cracked a little as she said it, making me think she did know what he did about it and it wasn't as fine as she wanted me to believe.

Her answers to the rest of the questions were all pretty generic, except she had been having more headaches than normal. I told Julie that what she was experiencing could have any number of causes, and we would have to do a thorough physical exam and then probably some simple testing. I stepped out of the exam room while she got ready.

Everything she had told me seemed to point to depression as the most likely cause of what she was experiencing, but I knew two things. First, this would not be a diagnosis she would accept easily. Perfect people don't get depressed. Tell them it's cancer and they somehow find solace in the fact that at least they're not to blame. Depression still has a stigma attached to it, a sense that this is a result of weakness, their fault. It generates a lot of internal chatter about just picking yourself up by the bootstraps and "What do you have to be depressed over, anyway?" The better off the patient, the less obvious the external problems, the greater the volume of the self-incrimination.

The second thing I knew right away was that jumping to a diagnosis might make me the winner on the medical version of *Jeopardy,* but it wasn't likely to purchase much in the way of patient confidence. The truth is this: Nobody wants to be "obviously" anything. A simple answer is not what any of us are really looking for. It's insulting. We all want to be what, in fact, we are—unique and a bit complex and not so easy to figure out. Blurting out some self-assured diagnosis without going through the process is always risky, a lesson I learned early in my career from a woman, mid thirties like Julie, who came in with very similar symptoms. When I asked the question about any sources of stress in her life, she unloaded. In the last year, one son had been hospitalized four times; the other had drug charges pending against him and was suspended from school. She was in the middle of a messy divorce after her husband had revealed an ongoing affair. What he didn't know was that she had had an affair herself, which resulted in a pregnancy and a secret abortion. Lately she was fighting a constant tiredness, and since her sister had just been diagnosed with "low thyroid," she wanted her thyroid tested as well. After hearing that soap-opera plot for a life, if ever I was sure that I was ordering a useless test this was it, but I ordered it anyway. I was shocked when two days later the results came back demonstrating that the patient, besides everything else, also had a thyroid problem. Nothing substitutes for a thorough process.

Julie's physical exam was pretty much normal. After Julie was dressed, I sat down and reviewed the results of my exam.

"Julie, I don't know exactly what you've got going on here. It could be a lot of things. It could be something purely physical. A thyroid disorder maybe, or anemia. It could be some other metabolic problem, like diabetes. It's just not entirely clear. We can get a better idea with some testing that I think will lead us one way or another. If the tests all come back normal, then we might need to consider depression as one of the possibilities. But we'll talk more about that at the next visit, after we have some of the results back."

A week later Julie and I sat in my office reviewing her test results.

"Well, Julie, as I told you on the phone, the results from your blood tests look very good." And I went through the list of what she didn't have. Again, saying the words was important. No evidence of cancer, no thyroid problems, no diabetes, no anemia.

I watched as her initial relief clouded over with concern.

"Now," I said. "It's a funny thing when you think about it. How all this good news of what you don't have can feel like bad news because you're still left with your symptoms and no explanation." I could tell by her eyes that I had hit pretty close to where she was. She was fighting back some tears.

"I think you could be experiencing a clinical depression, Julie. This is not the same as the 'blues' or simply feeling down. It can happen to people who, at least on the surface, seem to have no reason to be depressed. It's depletion more than anything else. If the theory du jour is right, it's a depletion of some hormones in your brain, chemicals that mediate a sense of energy and well-being and need to be at certain levels in order to do their job. The level of these hormones can become too low for a lot of different reasons. Sometimes we're doing things to ourselves that make them low. Sometimes there's a family pattern."

I watched her as I kept going with a speech I had delivered a hundred times. She was engaged but cautious. I had a feeling this wasn't going to play well at home. But I think her own need was so intense that for once what everyone else would think was not the driving force.

"Julie, there are many treatments for depression," I continued, "many of which can be very effective. I'm sure you have heard about Prozac and medicines like it. They've gotten a lot of press because, frankly, they work. These medicines have made treating depression much easier, maybe too easy, because I don't think it's the only answer. There are lots of other things that can enhance the treatment, things like diet and exercise, your spiritual life, and counseling." I noticed her face tighten at the word *counseling*. I needed to drive home its importance, even if it meant giving her someone to blame if necessary.

"I can't stress this too strongly. We have to be sure we're addressing everything. Treating depression without engaging a therapist would be like treating your kid's ear infections over and over and over again without ever addressing the role of their allergies." The crow's-feet above her brow were still there. So much for logic, time to throw the trump card. "Julie, I don't prescribe antidepressants for anyone who's not involved in some kind of counseling relationship."

I could see she was still struggling. I was struggling too. She needed more than a textbook here. She needed another human being. I drew in a deep breath and decided to speak out of my own experience.

"We all have our stuff, Julie. Trust me on this one. Patterns and pain we drag along with us. Holes inside we try to fill, usually with the wrong things. Sometimes we've carried it around for so long we just get used to it, stop even noticing it. But it still has its impact."

I had her attention. The quality of her listening changed as I moved from lecture to storytelling. "No one arrives at adulthood unscathed. We've all got issues. I've been through counseling myself; I had my own stuff to figure out. I spent an awful lot of my life being whatever the next person wanted me to be, hardly aware that I was doing it. In some ways it worked for me . . . for a while. I told myself it was 'professional' and therefore okay. I took an emotional elevator up and down to whatever floor the next patient was on, but the problem was it wasn't my emotion. I was only mirroring theirs. It was inauthentic. I was performing, Julie, trying to live up to some composite image of what I thought they needed me to be. After a while I couldn't even tell you what I was really feeling, other than maybe numb. Sometimes it takes an objective outsider we can be honest with to help us sort through stuff like that."

I held my breath and watched her watching me. I had crossed a line, and I wasn't sure how she would respond. Maybe she was thinking I was one of those pathetic "recently in counseling" psychoevangelists. Maybe she didn't want to hear anyone else's story. Maybe she didn't even buy the diagnosis. There were a few moments of silence, then her tense posture let down, relaxed a bit. I think she heard something in what I said that gave her a kind of permission. Almost whispering she said, "Do you have anyone you can recommend?"

I was relieved because I knew how big a hurdle this was for her. There would be many more to come, but getting over the first one is always the scariest. I went through an explanation of the medication and exactly how it worked, trying to put Serotonin Reuptake Inhibitor into a language someone without a neuroanatomy course could track. Julie left with the prescription and the card for the psychologist. We set up the next appointment for ten days later.

Thus began several months of seeing Julie regularly, every three to four weeks, monitoring her progress. I guess that's how doctors would refer to what was happening. The reality of it was that I think I cared for her in probably the best sense of that word. The visits always began with the usual questions about her medication: Was it effective? Was she having any side effects or problems? But eventually, we would get down to what she was confronting in counseling right then, as if she needed to share it with one more person in order to crystallize it. I mostly listened to her, and that was probably at least as therapeutic as the antidepressants. Slowly at first, but steadily, I witnessed a quiet transformation take place, the changes all the more real because of their subtlety. Visit by visit, the persona faded and a real person started coming into focus. The more Julie tasted of reality, the more she wanted. Up until now it was as if she had only experienced pictures of real things but not the real things themselves. A picture of a home, a picture of a family, a picture of herself. But the pictures could no longer satisfy. She needed something with substance, something to grasp a hold of.

Julie came together in a haphazard way, like a jigsaw puzzle being worked on by several people at the same time. How each section fit together wasn't really clear till the end. After a couple months of therapy, she was able to talk about some of the pain of her background, things even her husband didn't know. Things I think she had been dying to say out loud her whole life. One traumatic event had shadowed her since she was eight years old, an episode of sexual abuse at the hands of a neighbor. It was a dark secret she had never revealed before, and it permeated her life with a stain she couldn't seem to wash away. She had no memory of a single day since it happened when she just felt clean. She began to trace its far-reaching impact on her life.

She was raised in a strict Catholic family, which when combined with her oldest-child status, accentuated her ingrained sense of responsibility and guilt. Her father was a cold and distant man who emphasized only one thing—achievement. Julie grew up bent on proving something. She met and married her husband while in college, and there was probably an element of escape to her early marriage. It was then that Julie began in earnest the construction of her self-contained safe and ideal world. She convinced herself she could do it, convinced herself that with enough of the right exterior trappings she could actually erase the feelings inside, or at least cover them up. But all the attention to the outside of her life ended up playing a cruel trick. Instead of setting the stage for something fulfilling and meaningful, the extravagant exterior only seemed to accentuate the poverty inside.

Her marriage became a means to an end. How much of that was her problem and how much was her husband's was never clear. One morning, with tears in her eyes she told me she was sure Cameron was involved with someone else. All the signs were there. She didn't know who or how serious it was, but she knew something was going on. It was the weight of that suspicion and all the "what if's" chained to it that had finally driven her into my office that first morning.

Another section of the puzzle was her faith. A neighbor had been after her for a year to come to a women's Bible study group, but Julie had artfully dodged it, coming up with one excuse after another. I thought there had to be a reason she was telling me about this, so I encouraged her to give it a try. "What are you afraid of Julie? I doubt they make first-time visitors handle any snakes. They probably save that for later." I think she took my sarcasm as a challenge and finally relented. In the group, sticking out like a sore thumb from the other Stepford wives, was a friend of her neighbor, an older single missionary lady, home from Central America for a year. This lady was a peculiar little saint, and from Julie's description it was hard to imagine anyone with whom Julie could have had less in common. And yet, they connected and found they shared a kindred kind of spirit. I think this lady was so out of context that it allowed Julie to drop her pretense and honestly seek the answers to her questions.

As far as her faith was concerned, Julie had a lot of unfinished business. She told me she had grown up believing in God and Jesus and heaven and hell, but that belief was really little more than accepting a group of facts, like believing George Washington was the first president or the Egyptians built the pyramids. It didn't diffuse in any practical way into her day-to-day life. The God she knew, she only knew of; there was nothing personal to the relationship. Jesus? He was some vague, sad friend of the masses, and probably not someone who, if he came to visit, you'd want to stick around very long. Again I listened and at times shared some of my own story, about my own struggles with faith and doubt and finding a God who I believed cared, cared deeply and personally.

A God who found a way to bless us in spite of our pain and inadequacies; indeed, maybe even through them. Julie listened to a lot of different voices, and somewhere over that next year she grew into a faith that was personal and substantial. In many ways it empowered and helped sustain the changes going on in her life. Stone by stone the pretend castle she had hidden in for so long came down, gradually being replaced by a more modest but real home.

To say her husband did not greet the changes in Julie with exuberance is a gross understatement. He liked his life the way it was. He could count on it. He could control it, or at least make himself believe he could. Cameron was intent on his home being just another well-ordered, predictable enterprise, but now there was an element of uncertainty. All he really looked for from Julie's treatment was a return to baseline, and it was becoming increasingly apparent that wasn't going to happen. Julie was thinking on her own. Julie was confronting. Julie was talking about things she had never talked about before—things that weren't a part of Cameron's tidy little world. Julie was breathing, maybe for the first time ever, and it was evident she was never going back to holding her breath. It all left her husband nervous, uncertain of the new rules and the location of the out of bounds. There is something comforting about even a dysfunctional system when it's familiar and predictable. Change that system, even for the better, and you see people running for cover. No matter how much better the changes might have been for Julie, Cameron couldn't quite see past the impact it had on his own world.

Though counseling was often difficult, and replacing the

pretend with reality was tough work, Julie began to experience the exhilaration that came from allowing herself to be incomplete and in process. For Julie, twenty-five years of pretending came screeching to a halt. No . . . actually that's wrong. I guess it didn't come screeching to a halt; it just sort of ran out of gas and coasted slowly to a stop. Julie couldn't go on playing a part that wasn't really her. It seemed to me that her turning point came with the revelation of the secret that she had so carefully guarded for so long. That revelation brought her face to face with an inescapable conclusion—she was wounded and incapable of bringing about her own healing. Maybe all of us carry around the same dark secret. In some ways I think of it as a kind of blessed wound. Without it, how long would we continue to travel alone, confident in the illusion of our own adequacy? When it was all over, if I contributed in any way to Julie's healing it was out of my white coat, as someone able to listen to that secret and personally affirm the truth of it.

About eighteen months after that first visit for depression, Julie came in to tell me that the next corporate move was in play, and they would be moving to Boston soon. The decision was a scary one. For the first time ever she and Cameron had actually talked about it, actually treated it as if they could say no. She was anxious about leaving. She had done things here she had never done before. She had laid down some roots and developed relationships. But I think she was convinced that if the marriage was to survive, she needed to support the move. She still loved her husband and held tightly to the hope that a day would come when he, too, would be able to break out of his own captivity. Who better to show him the way than a recent escapee? I hoped that he wasn't looking at the move as just an easy way out, though I think deep down he might have secretly hoped that all the turmoil would just fade away in the relocation. It made me wonder what else he might be hoping would fade away with the move.

Julie came into the office for a final visit, more to say good-bye than anything else. When we had finished with all the business about transferring records and getting prescriptions filled, she turned to me and said something that I didn't quite know how to respond to. At the time, I didn't know whether to take it as an insult or one of the highest compliments I'd ever been paid. "You know, Dr. Judge, I'm really worried about something. I'm worried about finding another doctor. I've never been able to talk to a doctor like I've been able to talk to you." She paused a moment and then added, almost as an afterthought, "It's almost like you're not a doctor at all."

For some reason it stung a little bit when she said it. Maybe that's because no doctor really wants to hear he doesn't act like a doctor. Unless of course it's because he's acting like something more than a doctor—something more like a human being.

POSTSCRIPT

Several months after Julie moved to Boston I saw her counselor at a party. The counselor said she had heard from Julie just that week' and Julie said to be sure to say hello and let me know how she was doing. They had settled into a new home. The kids were adjusting well. She had already found another neighborhood Bible study. Her husband had finally agreed to go to counseling with her. He was reluctant and Julie didn't know exactly where their relationship was headed, but she was hopeful. It was a step in the right direction. She seemed confident that one way or another it would end up all right, and I had to agree. Sometimes all right can be a lot better than perfect.

NATHAN

The plane lurched and tipped wildly as we began our descent into Durham. It had been a rough ride. The "fasten your seat belt" sign had been on since our departure from Chicago. Hurricane Fran stood paused off the North Carolina coast, just about ready to make landfall, and the projected course put it directly over Raleigh-Durham within the next six hours.

The captain's voice crackled over the speakers.

"We apologize for all the turbulence, ladies and gentlemen. As you know we've got a little lady named Fran . . . sitting just off the coast, kicking up quite a stir. The airport at Raleigh-Durham is still open at this point . . . so we're going to make one attempt at landing. If we don't make it . . . we'll go on to Charlotte."

If we don't make it?! I thought to myself. *Is he kidding? I want to hear something a little more confident than "if we don't make it." Just exactly how do you measure "not making it"?* I wondered how close you get to the ground before you decide you're not going to "make it." The woman next to me was white-knuckling it, hands gripping the armrests, eyes focused straight ahead, mumbling. I couldn't quite make out whether it was her last confession or the text off the crash-landing instruction card from the seat back in front of her.

The plane pitched and yawed, then would even out for a couple of seconds, then seemed to drop out from under us, as if we were in free fall for 500 feet or so before going through the whole thing all over again. Gray clouds as close as your next breath streamed by the window. I could see nothing of the earth below. As we descended through the mist, I found myself staring out the window, caught up in my ongoing "through the clouds" fantasy. It was the upside-down one, where once we pass through the shroud it is the world below the clouds that is perpetually blue and at peace. A new world without problems, where everything is clear and the sun always shines and children didn't get sick. Especially the ones you know and love.

I looked again out the window and could see reality beginning to appear. As the mist thinned you could make out the dusk-darkened woods surrounding Raleigh-Durham. The winds must have momentarily calmed because the plane stabilized, and in what seemed like seconds we were plunked down hard onto the runway at the airport. The passengers broke out in spontaneous applause when the plane touched down. "Mumbles" next to me let go of the armrests (hers and mine) and started to breathe again. I myself fought a vague sense of disappointment; the bright carefree world my imagination hoped for had once again failed to appear. Maybe next time. The airport was deserted and eerie; ours was the last flight allowed in that night. I stepped out of the terminal into a gray, bleak world, knowing I was only trading one storm for another.

I was on my way to the Duke University Medical Center, not as a doctor, but as an uncle and brother and son. My thirteen- year-old nephew, Nathan, was scheduled for a complex brain surgery. My parents were already there at the hospital with him. My sister, Debbie, had left that morning to put some things together at home in preparation for spending the first postop week with her son. Her husband, Lucky, would arrive the next day. More than anything else I was here to just be with—with Nathan and my sister and her husband and my parents. I could feel a palpable tension building inside me, the product of the gap that stood between my hopes and fears. In one way or another I think we all wondered if we weren't approaching the end of the long and terrible journey that was Nathan's illness.

When he was about eleven years old, Nathan spontaneously developed seizures. The seizures were the "temporal lobe" variety, meaning there was no falling to the ground or jerking around. With his seizures Nathan would simply zone out for thirty to sixty seconds. They were more like short quiet journeys to someplace else. When he came out of them, he might drool or yawn or experience a facial twitch or just be really tired, unaware that a minute of life had just been stolen from him. At first the seizures were occasional, but soon they occurred multiple times each day, playing havoc with school and just about everything else in his life. Medication was prescribed, but wasn't very effective. As the amount and number of medications kept ratcheting up with the seizures' increasing frequency, a tragic Catch-22 developed: the medicines only converted Nathan from one kind of zombie to another. The source of the seizures remained elusive. CAT scans and MRIs and PET scans showed little more than a small area of what looked like scar tissue on one side of Nathan's brain.

Nathan had worked his way through several epilepsy experts, finally ending up at the Duke University Medical Center, which was several hours from his home. With more and more medicines resulting in less and less control of his seizures, a hard decision was made about a year after the seizures had begun. The doctors elected to do an open-brain biopsy to see if there was something they were missing in all the other tests.

Nathan's dad called us right after surgery. I think my sister couldn't make herself say the words. The scene at our home that day remains a terrible black-and-white snapshot I can't get out of my mind. I still remember where I sat, my wife and daughters there with me in the bedroom, the sun flooding in uninvited through the bedroom window. I was overwhelmed with a smothering helplessness as I heard my brother-in-law crying on the phone, struggling to say the words, as if saying the word *cancer* somehow gave it a greater reality. He was being bombarded with all the possibilities that yawned up in front of his son, in front of him.

Nathan had brain cancer of the most severe and complicated type. A many-tentacled tumor, not easily identifiable on scans, was working its way throughout one side of his brain. The tumor was inoperable. Five-year survival was almost unheard of. Chemotherapy and radiation therapy would need to begin at once, but were unpredictable and dangerous and would, at best, only slow it down. The seizures might never be controlled. I was numb for one brief moment after I hung up the phone. And then the tears began to flow and, as if I were the only one on earth, I began to cry as hard as I have ever cried. My wife and daughters were in the room and stood watching me. It was something they had never seen before.

Debbie and Lucky held their son's hand and walked with him into a world of chemotherapy and radiation treatments and fevers and midnight hospital vigils and the strain of trying to work life and their three other children around all of this. Recurrent nights of wondering what was being accomplished. Were they prolonging his life or his suffering? We all watched as Nathan, despite all that was being done, day by day lost more and more ground. He slept sixteen to twenty hours a day, and no one could sort out what part was played by the ongoing seizures or the side effects of an ever-increasing pharmacy of medications or the relentless progress of the cancer.

My view was from a distance, and it made me feel small and impotent and paralyzed. There was a part of me that wanted to take over, to somehow get in there and direct the cast of thousands that had become part of their lives. Radiation therapists and neurosurgeons and pediatric neurologists and oncologists and physical therapists. But I was a thousand miles away. It was impossible. I was caught wishing in a way for ignorance, because knowing too much only made things harder for me. If I checked up too much, I felt like I was diminishing his parents' ability to care for him. If I stood back too far, it felt as if I wasn't doing enough. So I settled into a nebulous limbo, listening to each report as it came in, trying hard to find something encouraging in it, and prayed.

Nathan was amazing through it all. He never complained. Never. He went from one doctor to the next, one medication to the next, one procedure to the next, as if this was the usual life of all twelve-year-old boys. And in between he managed to inject steady doses of Spiderman and Nerf guns and Ninja Turtles. There was no evidence that he ever felt sorry for himself. Of all the blessings that came along with his illness, Nathan's attitude was chief among them.

And there were, for sure, a thousand other blessings that came along with this curse. Big ones and small ones, planned ones and spontaneous ones. Like the woman, three towns over, herself a survivor of a brain tumor, who showed up at my sister's door one day with two gifts: a plate full of brownies and her own hopeful story. She sat with Debbie and Nathan and was, for them, a kind of living testimony, giving them enough hope to make it through that day. Friends from school and church rallied around them and showed a love comprised of flesh and words that demonstrated the power of real community. These things got them through—plus their faith and the blessing that comes with not being able to see too far down the road.

The relentless onslaught of the seizures kept coming, despite all the treatment. No amount of hope or wishful thinking could deny the fact that Nathan was deteriorating. No one knew what was going to take him first—the tumor or the treatment or an infection or some complication from the seizures. Hope was getting progressively harder to hold on to.

Nathan's medical team decided there was a chance that

a radical procedure could at least enhance the quality of Nathan's life, even if that was likely to be short. They could make a map of the electrical activity of Nathan's brain, place a grid over the general area they thought the seizures were coming from, and if the seizure source was localized, they could actually remove that part of the brain. This would hopefully eliminate the seizures and the need for medications. The complexity and the risk and the delicateness were almost incalculable. If the source of the seizure activity lay too close to an essential area, like the speech or motor center, Nathan could end up paralyzed or unable to speak. But there seemed to be little else anyone could offer that would make Nathan's last days any better lived. His parents agonized over it. They had seen their son put through so much already with so little to show for it, but what he was doing right now was barely living. If there was a significant chance the surgery could free him from the fog he was lost in, even if only for a matter of months, it would be worth it.

Watching Debbie and Lucky in the midst of all this was awe-inspiring. A strength grew that overwhelmed me. I had always seen my sister as quiet and delicate, someone who needed to be cared for. Her husband was her complementary side: in control, firmly directed, gifted with a strong sense of who he was. He seemed to walk through life free of fear, more sure than the next guy. But something was happening—they were trading roles, reaching down inside to find and develop within themselves what they needed to be for that time. Debbie was becoming very assertive in her own gracious style. She had educated herself well about

Nathan's medicines and treatments, about what complications to look for and what needed to happen when. Debbie was taking care. It was a mother's strength, something powerful I had never seen in her before. It was humbling. Lucky, on the other hand, was softening, developing a gentleness and tenderness that was strong all by itself. Suffering sometimes brings with it certain gifts. Qualities and strengths that are beyond value or measure, available only to those who have walked through suffering's gate. Yet I am sure, in our most intimate and private moments, if any of us were given the chance to walk away from the suffering, even if it meant leaving the new strength and wonder and faith with it, most of us would still choose the easier path. Maybe that's why the choice is so often not ours to make.

There were certainly no options as far as Nathan's suffering was concerned. His fate seemed sealed. Gradually we had all started talking in terms of making whatever time was left count. That was what this whole next step was about, and it required an immense amount of courage to take it. Not everyone thought it was the best choice. I knew my parents weren't excited about any more procedures. They were the soft side of the equation. Hadn't he suffered enough? They had seen so many things do so little good. They wanted a guarantee. They had their own pain to deal with, the pain that comes with feeling powerless. All they could see was one more operation, one more painful recovery. They just wanted to see his suffering end. I wonder if it would have been somehow easier if Nathan had complained, if he would have screamed bloody murder. It might have given voice to the hurting child inside all the rest of us.

I picked up my rental car and drove the ten miles into town, lost in the anticipation. I had an assignment from my wife and the therapist I was seeing—to keep current with what was going on inside me. To identify and feel what I was feeling as I was feeling it. Doesn't sound like a tough assignment, but for me it was mammoth because I was the king of delayed emotion. I had gone through most of my life with the basic assumption that it didn't matter what I felt because feeling one way or another wasn't going to change anything. "Just buck up" was a credo I had carried with me since childhood. In almost any situation I had learned to pick up the other person's emotional signal, strengthen it, and bounce it back to them. But it was inauthentic because it wasn't how I felt. Most of the time I couldn't tell you how I felt. So I sat there, struggling with the assignment to be me, not some image of what I thought a son or brother or uncle needed to be. It was my own new frontier, and I didn't know if I would be any good at it. As I drove toward town, there was a jumble of different emotions tumbling randomly inside. Like clothes in the dryer, first one would show itself at the window then another, with no reasonable link between them. My emotions right then were mostly differ-ent shades of fear. Fear for Nathan, fear of the unknown, fear of tomorrow, of what the strain of it all would leave when it was all over, as if it would ever be all over. I had seen tragedy bring some families together and tear others apart. Some strains build, others destroy. Our family's jury was still out.

We were all settling into our own emotional places. Each with its own nuance, its own particular shade. With my dad it was anger; with my mother it was fear; with me it was the inexpressible sadness of it all. A sadness that seemed almost cruel. In view of what was going on, I was torn between the obligation to defend God and the need to accuse him.

I met my dad in the hotel lobby, and as I checked in, he stood beside me giving instructions to both the clerk and me. Here I was, forty-three years old, and he still felt the need to take care of me. Before it had only grated on me. But now, for some reason, I could see a tenderness to it, a sweetness. And for once I didn't respond like a hacked-off thirteen-year-old. For once, it felt good. We walked through the hospital's parking garage and down the street together to the entrance.

Walking into Nathan's room felt like stepping into a tiny chapel. There was a surreal quality to the scene. The dim fluorescent hospital lighting. My mother sitting beside his bed looking tense and grim. Everyone talking in hushed tones. I embraced my mother, and we held one another that extra moment we both needed to grasp something familiar and loved, something anchored and safe.

"I'm so glad you made it. I was worried with the hurricane that they'd cancel your flight. How was it?" she asked.

"Bumpy, not that bad." My mother had a gross fear of flying. No sense going into the details. "It's getting bad outside though; the wind is really starting to blow."

We both stood looking at Nathan, my dad looking at us. Nathan was now thirteen. He hadn't eaten well for more than a year, despite tube feedings and IVs and every possible attempt to get him to do so. He was thin and pasty and emaciated. The hair that was just starting to return after the chemotherapy had been shaved. Multicolored tiny electrical wires fed up from his head and into a sort of stocking cap. They then ran into a single twenty-foot cable attached to a monitor the size of a small bookcase. There was a video camera focused on him that automatically recorded when the machine detected any seizure activity. Nathan was fogged in. A combination of medicines and the mapping procedure had placed him in a perpetual twilight.

"It's Uncle Jimmy, Nathan. I'm here."

He smiled with only a partial recognition, but then slipped back into his restless fitful sleep.

Keep fighting, Nathan, just keep fighting, was all I could think.

"How's he been, Mom?" I asked.

"Oh, he's doing okay. Aren't you, Nate?" she said, her hand stroking the sides of his face. "Really restless. I don't think he likes all those wires attached to his head. That dumb machine over there keeps going off all the time," she said.

The machine automatically recorded his brain-wave pattern every time he had a seizure. It kept going off because the seizures were almost continuous.

"Listen, why don't I sit here with him for a while," my dad broke in. "You and your mom take a break and go down to the cafeteria. She needs to get out of this room."

My mother and I wandered the cavernous hallways, which all seemed to be in the middle of some kind of reconstruction, and found our way to the cafeteria. It was about eight o'clock at night and it was pretty empty. We found a quiet corner and between sips of our drinks began to talk.

"How are you doing, Mom? You holding up okay?" She began to tear up right away. She needed to talk, I could tell. The pace of her speech was fast, almost panicked, as if there wasn't going to be time enough to say everything that needed to be said.

"I don't know. I just don't know if what we're doing here is right. How is this going to help? It's killing us all. I'm just so worried about your father. You know him, Jimmy; he gets so angry. But it's only because he cares so much. I'm afraid he's going to drive Debbie away with it. I tell him to just be quiet. Nathan's their son, we have to support what they're doing, but it's tearing your dad up inside. Sometimes I think it would be easier if we weren't so close, if we just moved away."

She paused a moment and then looked at me, almost afraid to say the words. "I'd do anything to stop this. Why does it have to be him? It should be me. I've lived a good long life. You know I'd change places in a minute. I've begged God to take me and let Nathan live." She was wiping away the tears with her napkin.

Her questions were questions only God could answer, questions of the heart; but there was release for her in just speaking them, as if speaking them let off some of the steam that was building inside. I reached across the table and held her hand.

She continued, her voice lowered. "There are times when I think it would just be easier if it was all over. But, Jimmy, I tell you, if Nathan dies I don't know what it's going to do to your dad."

She was crying and wiping her eyes through it all. It was

something I hadn't seen very often. My mother was the strong one. She had spent her childhood in Liverpool during World War II, running to bomb shelters, worrying about food, worrying about whether her younger siblings and mother had made it to a shelter or whether her dad or three older brothers would ever come home from the war. One of them didn't. Those years left their mark, and she walked away from them with a gift and a limp. The gift was the strength that comes from being a survivor, the confidence that nothing the world could throw at her would ever compare to what she had already experienced. The limp was her struggle with trusting, a sort of ever-present fear of what could be sitting around the next bend in the road. The knowledge that your whole world could be turned upside down. I was thinking about what she said. It was only the pain talking. It wouldn't be easier if they were far away; I could personally vouch for that. And it wasn't going to be easier when Nathan died. That is a lie we told ourselves to cut the pain, our search for the silver lining that didn't exist. Death may bring a certain peace for a suffering loved one, but it only opens a new dark chapter for those left behind. I had seen too many families standing on the other side, devastated with the realization that sick or suffering, simply holding on to life brings a comfort all its own.

I knew what she meant about the impact on my dad. Nathan was his second chance. There was a lot about his own kids that my father had missed. Travel and the '50s and all the baggage from his own motherless traumatic childhood had kept him emotionally separated from us. A typical night at my house growing up looked like this: there was Mom, as much friend as mother, sitting with the three kids laughing, watching TV, and then there was Dad—just four feet away, but always doing something else, in a world of his own, out of reach. My brother and sister and I made up stories as to why he wasn't there. My own story had a stiff dose of narcissistic self-accusation. Somehow it was my fault. There was something about me that kept him away. I took that story with me into adolescence and beyond. But I think most of life's answers are simple ones, and more than anything else, I think our problem was timing. It was simply off. Just when Dad wanted to draw closer, I was putting distance between us. Maybe to give support to the feelings inside. Maybe I had just found a way of punishing him.

No one stays the same. Everyone changes, with or without our permission. By the time Nathan arrived and my parents had moved within ten miles of my sister and her family, I think my father had become a different person. Nathan, from the beginning, had a gentleness and forgiveness about him that cast a wide net, wide enough certainly to capture my father's heart. He was the fair-haired child, a total boy surrounded by three sisters, who came with an unabashedly free need to just hang with the guys. From the earliest age, whenever we came to visit, Nathan would grab me by the hand and lead me to his room and show me his latest collection of action heroes or Spiderman comics. From his point of view, his uncle had come expressly to see him and be with him and that was all there was to it. Nathan had the gift of focus. When you were with him, there was nothing else in the world besides the two of you, and he shared this gift with my dad. They did all the things grandfathers and grandsons do: fishing and hiking and a lot of unstructured time together. The raw material of relationship.

I almost resented Nathan at times. Watching my dad with him could be painful. I stood at the edge watching them and found myself wanting to crash the party. I was jealous of Nathan's ability to just say what he needed. "Hey, come with me. I've got something to show you." I still couldn't say those words. The best I could do was to express my needs tangentially, by the way. Direct rejection was too much to be risked. It would be easier if I could tell myself the other person simply hadn't gotten the message. I don't believe Nathan ever saw rejection as even the remotest possibility. There was a part of me that was glad my father was working out a form of redemption with him. There was another part of me that wanted to scream, "Not fair!" Maybe in secret I was content to have the focus off of us, because if I was honest, I would have to admit that it wasn't my father keeping distance between us any longer. It was me. It was that stupid wounded adolescent I couldn't let go of.

"You need to do just like you're doing now, Mom. You have to talk about it. Those emotions are overpowering. And they always find their way out." I listened to myself and winced at the words; I sounded like some cheap psychologist. I tried again.

"There's enough pain to go around right now. Deb and Lucky have their brand; you and Dad have yours; I've got mine. We have to all take a lesson from Nathan. We all need to put on some courage and be real and tell each other when we're hurting and what we're afraid of and just hold on and pray we weather this with some kind of grace and strength."

I reached across the table and held her hand. It felt strange to be in the parental comforting role, but the border between parent and child had blurred. For a moment we were just two frightened travelers, caught in the same storm.

We walked slowly back up to the room and found my dad leaning over Nathan, gently dabbing away some drool from the corner of his mouth. I choked on the emotion. We sat together and talked of other things for a while, anything other than the tragedy at hand. It was a temporary but necessary diversion. We talked about my girls and our home and my new role at the clinic. I had taken on a significant administrative role, flying to various cities in a management/consultant position. It was a new world of big business and corporate jets and million-dollar budgets. On one level it sounded important but it all stood in stark contrast to the things that really mattered right now, like each other and the boy lying in the bed. Achievement was one of the few ways I had ever managed to get my father's attention. It still worked and, as always, it felt both good and bad. Like winning something you didn't deserve.

"I'll stay with him for a while. You and your dad go on down to the cafeteria."

I felt the usual tightness in my chest. "You and your dad . . ."

We walked slowly down the hall, not doing a whole lot of talking. We were both tired. I got a root beer and we sat at the same table where I had sat with my mother. I waited for it to start. It didn't take long.

He started in on how he didn't think this was the right thing to do, about the doctors not really knowing whether this was going to work, about how they had missed the diagnosis for a year, about how Nathan could be a vegetable, about being pushed around, about how wrong it was to be cutting a child's brain. It was an eruption more than anything else, an eruption that needed to happen. But in the middle of it all, a small miracle occurred. I sat watching him, and instead of concentrating on the words and feeling some necessity to correct or defend, I concentrated on his face and saw in it another message. He was in deep pain and he was frightened. What he wanted more than anything else was a guarantee. He wanted some kind of control over this awful thing; he wanted to be more than a spectator. He wanted what no one could give him.

I looked at him across the table and said, "It hurts us all to have to watch it. All we can hope is that there is some kind of wisdom, some kind of love behind it all. Something we can't see right now. And pray to God for enough strength."

"This isn't God. Why, if I thought God did this to Nathan, I'd . . . I'd . . . I'd want no part of a God like that, a God who could do this to a little boy." He was wiping his eyes.

I paused a moment and for once didn't feel a need to come to the defense.

"There are some answers that don't come when you want them, Dad. I think we end up living out most of our lives somewhere between the question and the answer. I don't know, maybe at its heart, that's what faith is all about."

He looked at me and something connected. We were both quiet for a moment, and in the time that followed we talked to each other, really talked and listened and were just there with each other. We kept talking the whole way back up to Nathan's room.

By this time the outer edge of the hurricane had arrived and the rain was beating almost horizontally against the long and narrow window in Nathan's room. The three of us argued about who would stay there with Nathan that night and my mom finally prevailed and sent the two men back across to the hotel. The rain pretty well soaked us and after hugging my dad good night I went up to my room. I stood there in the dark before getting into bed and watched the storm lashing the world outside. The trees bent and swirled in the winds that seemed to come from every direction at once, howling and screeching. Streetlights swayed in the tempest, making the world outside look as if it were caught up in a frantic voodoo dance. I lay back on the bed and fell fast asleep.

The next morning the hurricane had departed, leaving the city crippled. Hundreds of trees were down. Most of the city had no power. The hospital was working on its own emergency generators. Nathan had experienced an equally bad night. He had been increasingly restless and spiked a temperature in the middle of the night. There were chest x-rays and blood tests, none of which revealed very much. His temperature was now coming down again. About ten o'clock that morning Nathan's dad, Lucky, arrived, somehow getting through despite the aftermath of the storm. We sent my mother and dad back to the hotel for a much-needed nap. Neither of them had gotten much sleep.

As Lucky and I sat on opposite sides of Nathan's bed, we began to talk. All of the walls that keep two men from talking about how they really feel seemed to have blown away with the storm. We talked about Nathan and the tragedy of it all. We talked about the plain old waste and sadness. We talked about my parents and how they were reacting. As we talked, I found myself describing how I felt inside. My own loss, my own pain in watching my parents, my own struggle with believing there was a divinity in it all. And as I did tears ran down my cheeks, and I felt no need to wipe them away. They were simply a part of what I was feeling, nonverbal evidence of what was inside. Lucky had a strength and wisdom that carried both of us that morning. He wasn't denying his own pain; he didn't pretend it wasn't killing him. He had simply cried enough tears for now. But he was holding on to something, or it held on to him. Faith that let him see beyond the daily tragedy and kept hope alive. Maybe not hope for some miraculous healing, but hope that he and my sister and their other children and Nathan and all the rest of us would make it through this to some other side.

In some ways it was already happening. Nathan was bringing out the best in all of us. The last twenty-four hours had demonstrated that. We were all working hard at taking care of one another. I had flown in just to be with them, my dad at the hotel, my mom spending the night so we could sleep, my brother-in-law, of all things, comforting me. It reminded me of what an old Irish saint had said at the end of a book I had just finished:

To lend each other a hand when falling . . .

Perhaps that's the only work that matters in the end.

POSTSCRIPT

Nathan underwent the surgery and within a few days was back to shooting his Nerf gun at the nurses. For several weeks it looked as if the seizure activity was reduced, but two months later it was back to where it had been before the surgery. About this same time his parents went to see a neuro-surgical specialist at Johns Hopkins in Baltimore. His specialty was an even more radical procedure for children with unrelenting seizures—the removal of one entire half of a child's brain. Children have the capacity to transfer brain functions from one side of the brain to the other, something adults cannot do. The procedure had been done successfully with hundreds of children with intractable seizures but had never been performed on anyone with cancer. The other complication was Nathan's age. The rerouting of function happened most easily with younger children. Debbie and Lucky were faced with one more terrible decision. On the one hand was a future where Nathan would just sleep his way slowly toward certain death. On the other was the likelihood that with this at least the seizures would be gone. But what would go with them? They made the only decision a parent could.

Nathan was operated on two years ago, and the entire right half of his brain was removed. The tissue samples revealed no evidence of any residual cancer. He recuperated well, and to everyone's relief it was the same old Nathan who woke up after the operation, wanting his action videos within the first week. He has never had another seizure. He is off all medications. He just started regular high school classes. He has a little motor weakness on one side but walks independently. His biggest challenge is regaining his speech ability, though he has no problem getting his message across.

No one is saying the word *cure;* no one dares. But it is a word that hangs in the air like hope.

EPILOGUE

There were always going to be ten chapters, ten stories. I don't really know why. I suppose it was nothing more compelling than the attraction of an even number. But when I finished the ninth story and reread the book, I realized that I had already inadvertently told a tenth story—my story—woven in and out of the others.

During my last five years of private practice I took on more and more leadership and administrative responsibilities, dwindling down my actual patient-care time to a token half day a week. Probably trying to convince myself, more than anyone else, that I had not become a suit. As with most decisions in life, I was both pushed and pulled. What pushed me out of patient care was only evident to me years later. What pulled me was the gravitational force of something new—new skills and new words and new places. I think I was also looking for something new to conquer, something requiring just a little less heart. And mixed with it all was an unhealthy dose of being sure I was the only one who could protect our clinic from the forces of change that boiled all around us.

As the result of multiple mergers and the acquisition of various clinics, my responsibilities became national in scope.

Many weeks I spent three days or more in other states. But as the newness and excitement wore off, it became apparent that coming to work was becoming less and less fulfilling. I looked at what I was doing every day and had a hard time passing the "so what?" test. I saw those with whom I spent my days, how little we had in common, and the leadership that placed patient care a distant second to the bottom line. The cost to my soul was mounting. When the opportunity came with the final merger for me to take a year's severance and leave, I decided it was time to go.

When I thought about a year to do as I wished, there was only one option. Writing. There were stories pounding on the door of my soul. The patient stories I had told and retold over the years. The ones I couldn't stop telling. The tales from my personal diary. It was a great challenge—to write them, to write them well, the best I could, and in so doing, maybe honor them, maybe complete them. If nothing else, at least turn their pulsating volume down in my head.

About halfway through that year I came to understand two truths that had somehow been misplaced among the clutter that was my life. First, the reason these stories had such sway over my soul was that they weren't just passive portrayals of events that had happened to someone else. They were, in essence, my story as well. As much as anyone else, I was the one changed with each encounter, with each touch. And second, the truth that the personal patient encounter gave me much more than an identity; in some ways, it gave me life. It was what I loved to do more than anything else.

At the end of that year, when it came time to look for a "real job," I first looked at positions that focused on my administrative background. But I found myself always asking the same question: "Can I also see patients?" As the time to decide on each opportunity drew near, I kept pulling my hat out of the ring at the last minute. Then a call came for a position the recruiter was sure I wouldn't be interested in but maybe I knew someone who would. It was at a small primary-care office associated with a well-known medical center/medical school not far away. Administrative responsibilities would be minimal; it was really more patient care than anything else, and oh by the way, there was an expectation to teach one day a week at the medical school. Sometimes it's not only in youth that the door opens just a crack and lets the future in. It can happen to middle-aged people as well. I interviewed, and while walking through the medical school I felt a warm resonance inside my soul. This was the place.

And so today, besides the medical practice, I teach medical students each week. What I teach them mostly is the art of medicine. That there is something beyond the detective work, beyond the technique. Like how to talk to a patient, how to make them feel comfortable. How your voice and your pace of speech and whether you sit or stand, your eye contact, all work together to convey a message—they are not a number or a case, but a human being. A message of caring that patients today are ever more desperate to hear. My challenge is to teach my students that they, in the final analysis, are the therapeutic instruments. And even more improbably, that the healing can go in both directions.

I continue to write. It is a part of who I am. And there are so many more stories waiting to be told.

D R. JAMES JUDGE is a practicing physician who teaches at Loyola's Stritch School of Medicine in Chicago. After more than twenty years of practicing medicine, the tension between medicine's science and art, its knowledge and compassion, its head and heart continues to challenge him every day.

He and his wife, Cindy, live in Wheaton, Illinois, with their three daughters.